DIABETES IN WOMEN

PUBLIC HEALTH IN THE 21ST CENTURY

Additional books in this series can be found on Nova's website under the Series tab.

Additional E-books in this series can be found on Nova's website under the E-books tab.

PUBLIC HEALTH IN THE 21ST CENTURY

DIABETES IN WOMEN

ELIZA I. SWAHN
EDITOR

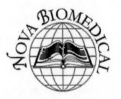

Nova Science Publishers, Inc.
New York

Library of Congress Cataloging-in-Publication Data
Available upon request

ISBN: 978-1-61668-692-5

Published by Nova Science Publishers, Inc. ✦ *New York*

Contents

Preface

Diabetes is a unique condition for women. When compared with men, women have a 50 percent greater risk of diabetic coma, a condition brought on by poorly controlled diabetes and lack of insulin. Women with diabetes have heart disease rates similar to men, but more women with diabetes die from a first heart attack than do men with diabetes. Diabetes also poses special challenges during pregnancy. This new book discusses and presents topical data on the effects of diabetes in women, such as: diabetes mellitus in pregnant women and birth outcomes, assessing bone condition in women with Type 2 diabetes, depression and cardiovascular disease in women with diabetes, and others.

Chapter I - The aims of this review are (i) to differentiate the adverse birth outcomes of pregnant women with type 1 (DM-1), type 2 (DM-2) and gestational diabetes mellitus (GDM) because these different types of DM were combined and/or confused frequently in previous studies, (ii) in the population-based Hungarian data to exclude the selection bias of the previously published hospital-based materials, and (iii) to check the efficacy of the recent special prenatal care of diabetic pregnant women introduced in Hungary during the 1980s in the prevention of adverse birth outcomes of diabetic pregnant women. Among adverse birth outcomes, the rate of preterm and postterm births, low and large birthweight of newborns, in addition the risk of structural birth defects, i.e. congenital abnormalities (CA) were estimated in the offspring of pregnant women with medically recorded DM-1, DM-2 and GDM compared the occurrence of different DM in pregnant women who had malformed fetuses/newborns (cases) and who delivered healthy babies (controls) in the population-based Hungarian Case-Control

Surveillance System of Congenital Abnormalities, 1980-1996. In the case group including 22,843 offspring, there were 79 (0.35%) pregnant women with DM-1, 77 (0.34%) pregnant women with DM-2 and 120 (0.53%) pregnant women with GDM. The control group comprised of 38,151 newborns, 88 (0.23%), 141 (0.37%) and 229 (0.60%) had pregnant women with DM-1, DM-2 and GDM. The mean gestational age at delivery was shorter in the newborns of pregnant women with DM-1 while longer in the newborns of pregnant women with DM-2. The mean birth weight was largest in the newborns of pregnant women with GDM followed by DM-1, while the mean birth weight in the group of DM-2 did not differ from the reference value. On the contrary the rate of low birthweight was not lower in babies born to mothers with GDM, than in the reference sample, and the larger mean birth weight associated with the higher (the highest) rate of low birthweight newborns in the group of DM-1. The rate of large birthweight newborns was the highest in the group of GDM. Thus these data indicate a higher risk of both small and large birthweight newborns in DM-1 and a higher risk of large birthweight newborns in the group of GDM. The total rate of cases with CA was higher only in the group of DM-1 (adjusted OR with 95% CI: 1.5, 1.1-2.0) due to 4 specific types/groups: isolated renal a/dysgenesis, obstructive CA of urinary tract, cardiovascular CAs and multiple CAs mainly caudal dysplasia sequence which had a higher risk in the offspring of pregnant women with DM-1. However, the risk of total CAs was lower in the study compared to the risk of previous studies and the DM-1 related spectrum of isolated CAs was also different (e.g. there was no higher risk of neural-tube defects) and these findings indicate that certain part of maternal teratogenic effect of DM-1 is preventable with appropriate periconceptional and prenatal care of diabetic women including folic acid supplementation. There was no higher risk of total CA in the offspring of pregnant women with DM-2 and GDM. In conclusion the different type of DM associates with different fetotoxic and teratogenic risk for their offspring and the recent specific prenatal care of diabetic pregnant women seems to be more effective in the reduction of DM related isolated CA than other adverse birth outcomes because a higher rate of both intrauterine fetal retardation and large babies were found in the newborns of pregnant women with DM-1 while large birthweight was recorded in the newborns of pregnant women with GDM. The major finding of our studies was that the recent special prenatal care of diabetic pregnant women including folic acid supplementation was able to reduce a significant part of maternal teratogenic effect of DM-1. Thus our study indicated first that folic acid supplementation is appropriate for the prevention of DM related isolated CAs.

Chapter II - Although bone mineral density (BMD) is considered as a gold standard for evaluating fracture risk in non-diabetic osteoporosis, accumulative evidence shows that patients with type 2 diabetes have high fracture rate in spite of the absence of BMD reduction, indicating that BMD is not sensitive enough to assess the risk of osteoporotic fractures in them. In addition, hyperglycemia itself is not associated with BMD or fracture risk, either. Therefore, the etiology of diabetes-related bone fragility and its diagnostic markers replacing BMD need to be explored. Advanced glycation end products (AGEs), which are produced by sequential nonenzymatic chemical glycoxidation of protein amino groups under hyperglycemia, accumulate in various tissues during normal aging, and may play a pivotal role in the development of complications including bone fragility in diabetic patients. Bone metabolism in type 2 diabetes is also affected by diabetes-related abnormality in hormonal actions of insulin and insulin-like growth factor-I (IGF-I). Our previous clinical studies have shown that serum levels of pentosidine, which is one of the well-known AGEs, as well as IGF-I could be clinically useful for assessing the risk of vertebral fractures in postmenopausal women with type 2 diabetes. On the other hand, recent animal experiments and clinical studies have indicated that osteocalcin, specifically produced by osteoblasts, acts as a hormone improving obesity and hyperglycemia, suggesting that bone metabolism and glucose/fat metabolism are etiologically related to each other. Several experiments have shown that adiponectin, one of the adipocytokines and a key mediator of visceral fat accumulation, has a stimulatory action on osteoblastogenesis and bone formation. We also found that serum adiponectin level was associated with serum osteocalcin in patients with type 2 diabetes in clinical studies. Thus, serum adiponectin may be useful for assessing not only glucose/fat metabolism but also bone metabolism including osteoblasts in diabetic patients.

Chapter III - Self management of diabetes is an essential component of diabetes care, and to achieve good self-care people with diabetes should be knowledgeable about the purpose and clinical utility of diagnostic tests and monitoring. In this study we sought to identify and describe women's attitudes to diabetes, their knowledge of diabetes, their self management behaviours, and their health outcomes and, to explore the interrelationship between these factors. The study involved analysis of survey data from 223 women aged 50-55 years, and 655 women aged 75-80 years participating in the Australian

Longitudinal Study on Women's Health, who reported having diabetes. Survey data included socio-demographic and health variables, type and duration of diabetes, level and frequency of diabetes care, knowledge, attitudes and self-care practices, and access to diabetes-related health services and diabetes education services. Most women expressed positive attitudes regarding their adjustment to having diabetes although a large proportion of women did not engage in appropriate behaviours and preventive activities. In general the women in both age groups had less than optimal levels of knowledge, although women who had attended a diabetes education centre had better knowledge scores. Better knowledge was correlated with better behaviours (in both age groups) and with better health outcomes (among older women). The results of the study indicate that, at a community level, there is a great need to improve knowledge and behaviours among the growing population of women with diabetes, particularly those with Type II diabetes and older people. The results also provide strong support for the work of diabetes education centres.

Chapter IV - Background. In contrast to ST elevation myocardial infarcts in non-ST-elevation myocardial infarction (NSTEMI) prognosis in women and men are equal and in unstable angina even in favour of women compared to men. Diabetes is common amongst patients admitted with NSTEMI, in particular in women as demonstrated by several clinical trials. Diabetic in comparison with non diabetic patients with NSTEMI in general have more clinical complications, increased mortality, longer in-hospital stay and increased management costs. However, the prognosis in diabetic women in comparison to their diabetic counterparts, diabetic and nondiabetic men with NSTEMI is less well known. Our aim was to evaluate and compare 30-day mortality between diabetic and nondiabetic women, diabetic women and diabetic and nondiabetic men with NSTEMI.

Patients and Methods: We retrospectively analysed all the records of patients discharged with the diagnosis NSTEMI during one year period. 415 patients, 181 women (mean age 71,2 ± 11,9 years), 234 men (mean age 64.8 ± 10.8 years) fullfilled the inclusion criteria, being rest chest pain, lasting up to 48 hours before addmission, ECG changes without ST-elevation, but with ST-depression and/or negative T wave and increase in Troponin T, estimated by immunochemical method (normal levels up to $0.1 \mu g/l$), suggesting the size of ischemic necrosis. The patients were treated by antiplatelet, anticoagulant therapy and percutaneous coronary intervention. During 30-day follow-up demographic data, in particular diabetes, and 30-day mortality were registered.

Results: Diabetes was observed in 24.3% of patients with NSTEMI. Between the genders there was a nonsignificant difference in the incidence of diabetes, being 22.8% in women and 25.7% in men. Mean admission troponin T level was $0.38 \pm 0.7\mu g/l$ and peak Troponin T $0.82 \pm 1.3\mu g/l$. There were nonsignificant differences in mean peak Troponin T levels between diabetic and nondiabetic patients ($0.81 \pm 1.6\mu g/l$ vs $0.8 \pm 1.2\mu g/l$), diabetic and nondiabetic women ($1.2 \pm 2.0\mu g/l$ vs $0.81 \pm 1.2\mu g/l$), diabetic women and nondiabetic men ($1.2 \pm 2.0\mu g/l$ vs $0.82 \pm 1.3\mu g/l$) and diabetic women and men ($1.2 \pm 2.0\mu g/l$ vs $0.56 \pm 0.9\mu g/l$). 30-day mortality of patients with NSTEMI was 4.3%. Any significant differences were observed in overall 30-day mortality between men and women (3.0% vs 9.3%), neither between diabetics and nondiabetics with NSTEMI (5.9% vs 3.8%), between diabetic and nondiabetic women (6.9% vs 5.5%), nondiabetic men and nondiabetic women (2.4% vs 5.5%) and between diabetic men and women (5.2% vs 6.9%).

Conclusion: 30-day mortality in diabetic women with NSTEMI is similar to nondiabetic patients with NSTEMI, either men or women.

Chapter V - The number of diabetic patients has been estimated to at least double during the next 30 years worldwide. Cardiovascular disease is the leading cause of death among patients with type 2 diabetes. The associations of type 2 diabetes and hyperglycemia with the risk of cardiovascular disease have been assessed by a number of prospective studies and the results are consistent. Patients with type 2 diabetes have a 2-4 times higher risk of coronary mortality than those without diabetes. Among middle-aged general population, men have 2 to 5 times higher risk of coronary heart disease than women. However, women with diabetes will loose their relative protection against coronary heart disease compared with men. In recent years, several studies compared the gender specific impact of diabetes and myocardial infarction at baseline on cardiovascular mortality. These studies found that both diabetes and myocardial infarction at baseline increased coronary mortality. In women, prior myocardial infarction at baseline confers a lower or the same risk on coronary mortality than prior diabetes does. The results of these studies have important implications for clinical practice that we need to consider carefully the treatment strategies on individual disease status, particularly type 2 diabetes in women, for future coronary heart disease risk.

Cardiovascular disease (CVD), especially coronary heart disease (CHD) and stroke, is the leading killer in western societies and its prevalence is also increasing dramatically in developing nations (1, 2). Preliminary mortality data show that CVD as an underlying cause of death accounted for 34.2% of all 2 425 900 deaths in 2006 or 1 of every 2.9 deaths in the United States (3). CHD caused about 1 of every 5 deaths in the United States in 2005(3). High blood pressure, smoking, dyslipidemia, overweight or obesity, physical inactivity, diabetes, chronic inflammation, hemostatic factors, psychosocial factors, perinatal conditions and several dietary factors are the main risk factors for CVD (3-6). There is a significant difference in CVD risk between sexes (7, 8). Among middle-aged people, men have 2- to 5-times higher CVD mortality rates than women (8). The sex difference in CVD mortality cannot be completely explained by abnormal levels of conventional CVD risk factors, such as high blood pressure, lipid abnormalities, smoking and obesity (8).

Diabetes is one of the fastest growing public health problems in both developing and developed countries (9). It has been estimated that the number of individuals with diabetes among adults 20 or more years of age will double from the current 171 million in 2000 to 366 million in 2030 (9). Much of the burden of diabetes is attributable to microvascular and macrovascular complications, such as retinopathy, nephropathy, CHD, and stroke. CVD accounts for more than 70% of total mortality among patients with type 2 diabetes (10). Epidemiological studies have indicated that patients with type 2 diabetes have a 2-4 times higher risk of CVD mortality than those without diabetes (11-13). The Framingham Study is the first one to point out that women with diabetes seem to lose their relative protection against CHD compared with men (14). The reason for the higher relative risk of CHD in diabetic women than in diabetic men is still unclear. In this chapter, we summarize current results regarding the role of type 2 diabetes on the risk of CHD among women.

Chapter VI - Diabetes and depression are both significant public health concerns for women. Depression is a risk factor for incident type 2 diabetes, and it also increases risk for poor diabetes outcomes. Research linking depression to health risks is limited in several important ways, particularly by common practices employed to measure depression. In this chapter we review evidence linking depression and diabetes in women, and describe limitations of the extant literature. We then review our own work that begins to address these limitations. We conclude with a review of the treatment literature and recommendations for addressing depression in women with diabetes.

In: Diabetes in Women   ISBN: 978-1-61668-692-5
Editor: Eliza I. Swahn, pp. 1-24   © 2010 Nova Science Publishers, Inc.

Chapter I

Diabetes Mellitus in Pregnant Women and Adverse Birth Outcomes

Andrew E. Czeizel[a], Nándor Ács[b] and Ferenc Bánhidy[b]*
[a]Foundation for the Community Control of Hereditary Diseases,
Budapest, Hungary
[b]Second Department of Obstetrics and Gynecology, Semmelweis
University, School of Medicine, Budapest, Hungary

Abstract

The aims of this review are (i) to differentiate the adverse birth
outcomes of pregnant women with type 1 (DM-1), type 2 (DM-2) and
gestational diabetes mellitus (GDM) because these different types of DM
were combined and/or confused frequently in previous studies, (ii) in the
population-based Hungarian data to exclude the selection bias of the
previously published hospital-based materials, and (iii) to check the
efficacy of the recent special prenatal care of diabetic pregnant women
introduced in Hungary during the 1980s in the prevention of adverse

---

[*] Corresponding author: 1026 Budapest, Törökvész lejtõ 32. Hungary
Tel: +36 1 3944 712, Fax: +36 1 3944 712
E-mail: czeizel@interware.hu

birth outcomes of diabetic pregnant women. Among adverse birth outcomes, the rate of preterm and postterm births, low and large birthweight of newborns, in addition the risk of structural birth defects, i.e. congenital abnormalities (CA) were estimated in the offspring of pregnant women with medically recorded DM-1, DM-2 and GDM compared the occurrence of different DM in pregnant women who had malformed fetuses/newborns (cases) and who delivered healthy babies (controls) in the population-based Hungarian Case-Control Surveillance System of Congenital Abnormalities, 1980-1996. In the case group including 22,843 offspring, there were 79 (0.35%) pregnant women with DM-1, 77 (0.34%) pregnant women with DM-2 and 120 (0.53%) pregnant women with GDM. The control group comprised of 38,151 newborns, 88 (0.23%), 141 (0.37%) and 229 (0.60%) had pregnant women with DM-1, DM-2 and GDM. The mean gestational age at delivery was shorter in the newborns of pregnant women with DM-1 while longer in the newborns of pregnant women with DM-2. The mean birth weight was largest in the newborns of pregnant women with GDM followed by DM-1, while the mean birth weight in the group of DM-2 did not differ from the reference value. On the contrary the rate of low birthweight was not lower in babies born to mothers with GDM, than in the reference sample, and the larger mean birth weight associated with the higher (the highest) rate of low birthweight newborns in the group of DM-1. The rate of large birthweight newborns was the highest in the group of GDM. Thus these data indicate a higher risk of both small and large birthweight newborns in DM-1 and a higher risk of large birthweight newborns in the group of GDM. The total rate of cases with CA was higher only in the group of DM-1 (adjusted OR with 95% CI: 1.5, 1.1-2.0) due to 4 specific types/groups: isolated renal a/dysgenesis, obstructive CA of urinary tract, cardiovascular CAs and multiple CAs mainly caudal dysplasia sequence which had a higher risk in the offspring of pregnant women with DM-1. However, the risk of total CAs was lower in the study compared to the risk of previous studies and the DM-1 related spectrum of isolated CAs was also different (e.g. there was no higher risk of neural-tube defects) and these findings indicate that certain part of maternal teratogenic effect of DM-1 is preventable with appropriate periconceptional and prenatal care of diabetic women including folic acid supplementation. There was no higher risk of total CA in the offspring of pregnant women with DM-2 and GDM. In conclusion the different type of DM associates with different fetotoxic and teratogenic risk for their offspring and the recent specific prenatal care of diabetic pregnant women seems to be more effective in the reduction of DM related isolated CA than other adverse birth outcomes because a higher rate of both intrauterine fetal retardation and large babies were found in the newborns of pregnant women with DM-1 while large birthweight was recorded in the newborns of pregnant women with GDM. The major finding of our studies was that the recent special prenatal care of diabetic pregnant women including folic acid supplementation was able to reduce a significant part of maternal teratogenic effect of DM-1. Thus our study indicated first that folic acid supplementation is appropriate for the prevention of DM related isolated CAs.

Introduction

The placenta is a highly potent endocrine organ producing steroid and protein hormones, therefore strongly influences maternal carbohydrate metabolism [32]. Glucose freely passes through the placenta, but maternal insulin does not. The fetus begins to produce insulin from the 11th gestational week. Permanent glucose oversupply to the fetus stimulates the fetal pancreatic islet cells to increase insulin production and it gradually induces their hypertrophy and hyperplasia.

The mean blood glucose in normal pregnancy is 5.0 to 5.6 mmol/L (90 to 100 mg/dl). The fasting blood glucose level sinks to 3.3 to 3.9 mmol/L (60 to 70 mg/dl) during the course of normal pregnancy. The postprandial blood glucose level in pregnancy elevated to 7.2 to 7.8 mmol/L (130 to 140 mg/dl) due to the result of placental anti-insulin hormones.

Glucose tolerance improves in normal early pregnancy due to the effect of human chorionic gonadotropin; however, there is a progressive decrease in glucose tolerance after the 20th gestational week associated with placental anti-insulin hormones.

Insulin secretion is increased during normal pregnancy with gestational age. However, the effect of insulin is enhanced by insulinotropic hormones before the 20th gestational week, but is decreased thereafter by the effect of anti-insulin hormones.

Thus the glucose homeostasis is changed in the direction of diabetes mellitus in normal pregnancy, therefore glucose tolerance gradually deteriorates for which reason pregnancy is often called "diabetogenic".

Diabetes mellitus (DM) is a common disease, recently with an increasing prevalence in childbearing age, therefore, in pregnant women as well.

The first level classification of DM differentiates 3 types:

Type 1 (DM-1)

Type 1 (DM-1) is a chronic autoimmune disease due to inadequate insulin production by the islet beta cells due to the interaction of genetic and environmental factors causing progressive islet cell destruction in the pancreas. These patients with low to absent insulin level and acute or subacute appearance of DM-1 symptoms need insulin treatment for life. The onset of DM-1 is predominantly under 30 years with a peak of 9 years (explaining its previous term: juvenile-onset DM or insulin dependent DM: IDDM); in general, in non-obese persons who are prone to ketosis.

Type 2 (DM-2)

Type 2 (DM-2) is a chronic disease arising from progressive tissue insulin resistance caused again by the interaction of genetic and environmental factors [29]. These patients with variable insulin level and in general slow appearance of symptoms need diet control and/or oral hypoglycemic drugs. The onset of DM-2 is predominantly over 30 years (explaining its previous term: adult-onset DM or non-insulin dependent DM: NIDDM), although the past 12-20 years have seen a dramatic increase in the prevalence of DM-2 in children and adolescents [41], commonly in obese (often central or masculine obesity type), however, ketosis is less likely. Insulin treatment may also be required later in these patients to control hyperglycemia.

Gestatiional DM (GDM)

Gestational DM (GDM) is defined as glucose intolerance of any degree that begins or is first recognized during pregnancy. This pregnancy complication occurs about 4% of pregnancies [5]. The explanation of GDM is the maternal tissue insulin resistance due to the drastic hormonal changes in pregnant women. GDM is similar to DM-2, thus most of them are a preclinical state of DM-2 with a later onset [24]. Pregnant women with GDM need medical nutritional therapy and insulin when necessary. Insulin treatment in GDM is primarily important for the fetus, thus insulin treatment is indicated when, despite diet, fasting blood glucose value repeatedly exceed 6.1 mmol/L (110 mg/dl) and in pregnant women with a mean blood glucose exceeding 7.2

mmol/l (130 mg/dl) even when the fasting blood glucose is below 6.1 mmol/L (110 mg/dl) [42]. Shortly after delivery, glucose homeostasis is restored to non-pregnancy levels, but affected women remain at high risk of developing DM-2, obesity and metabolic syndrome in the future [38].

DM and pregnancy "do not like" each other therefore DM is a "malignant" disease during pregnancy. On one hand pregnancy can modify the maternal DM because interprandial hypoglycemia becomes more severe parallel with the progress of pregnancy therefore the status of DM has become worse with the necessary change of treatment. On the other hand DM can cause pregnancy complications and adverse pregnancy/birth outcomes including birth defects. This dangerous interaction can be explained by the growing fetal glucose demand and the function of placenta with increasing level of diabetogen steroids and peptide hormones (estrogens, progesterone, and chorionic somatomammotropin). The increase of these hormonal levels results in a progressively rising tissue resistance to maternal insulin action. Thus the hypoglycemia is more severe between meals and at night in pregnant women therefore insulin production in the pancreas increases more than two-fold compared with non-pregnant level during feeding. However, the failure in the increase of pancreatic insulin output induces maternal and fetal hyperglycemia; therefore it is necessary to increase exogenous insulin treatment. Fetal hyperglycemia is followed by fetal hyperinsulinemia which is dangerous for fetal well-being and consequently fetal growth because promotes storage of excess nutrients and consequently macrosomia.

Macrosomia, i.e. high birth weight (above 4500 g or above the 90th percentile for gestational age) is caused mainly by fetal obesity due to fetal hyperinsulinemia particularly in the third trimester. Skeletal growth is largely unaffected. Fetal obesity is concentrated mainly in the truncal region thus the measurement of abdominal circumference by ultrasound after the 24th gestational week but mostly from the 32nd weeks can detect it [7]. High birth weight was found 3-fold higher in the newborn infants of diabetic pregnant women compared to normoglycemic control pregnant women [6], especially in females with underlying vascular diseases. Of course, macrosomia associates with a higher risk of birth injury, mainly shoulder dystocia and branchial plexus trauma. However, the weight of fetus/newborns of diabetic pregnant women generally is skewed in both sides of their distribution, thus, there is a higher risk of low and high birth weight newborns.

Thus low birthweight newborns, i.e. intrauterine growth retardation were also found in a significantly higher rate in diabetic pregnant women, particularly with vasculopathy (retinal, renal and heart complications), preeclampsia, and hypertension. Thus uteroplacental vasculopathy may be the common denominator in the origin of intrauterine growth retardation of fetuses in the pregnancy of diabetic women. This U-shaped higher risk is explained by the characteristics of diabetic pregnant women.

The risk of structural birth defects, i.e. congenital abnormalities (CAs) in the offspring of pregnant women with overt DM prior to conception was 4 to 8-fold higher [37]. This high risk is explained by the maternal teratogenic effect of DM because there is no higher risk of CA in the children of diabetic fathers, normoglycemic pregnant women and women with GDM if its onset was after the first trimester. Another important argument for the maternal teratogenic effect of DM i.e. "diabetic embryopathy" is that this maternal disease associated with specific isolated CAs [31, 4] and a specific multiple CA including characteristic component CAs, the so-called caudal dysplasia sequence [26, 39, 35, 34]. The primary CA of the caudal dysplasia sequence (its previous name was caudal regression syndrome) is the caudal region including the incomplete development of the sacrum (sometimes associated with the CA of the lumbar vertebrae as typical spina bifida aperta) and femoral head, renal a/dysgenesis, imperforate anus, and sometimes orofacial clefts. While the secondary consequences of the primary CAs are clubfoot, flexion and abduction deformity of hips, popliteal webs, in addition to urine and feces incontinence due to neurologic impairment of the distal spinal cord.

In addition the spectrum of maternal DM related CAs encompasses isolated neural-tube defects [30], cardiovascular CAs particularly transposition of the great vessels, double outlet right ventricle, and common truncus [22, 27], kidney CA (renal a/dysgenesis), CAs of the urinary tract, congenital limb deficiency (mainly the lack of femoral head), and CAs of the skeletal system, mainly CAs of spines [23, 28, 40].

The primary cause of maternal DM related CAs is hyperglycemia which may promote excessive formation of oxygen radicals in susceptible fetal organs and tissues which are inhibitors of prostacyclins [32]. The secondary consequence is the predominance of thromboxanes causing a disruption of the vascularization of embryonic organs.

There is a higher risk of neonatal morbidity (polycythemia, hyperviscosity, hypoglycemia, cardiomyopathy, respiratory distress syndrome, etc) and associated mortality of the infants of diabetic pregnant women [32] but this important topic is out of our experiences. The maternal complications of diabetic pregnant women (retinopathy, nephropathy, cardiovascular diseases, diabetic ketoacidosis) and the higher rate of fetal mortality, i.e. miscarriages due to poor glucose control [23] are also not discussed here. There are three aims of this review based on our previous studies [1-3]:

1. The differentiation of adverse birth outcomes of pregnant women with DM-1, DM-2 and GDM because these different types of DM were combined and/or confused frequently in previous studies.
2. Our Hungarian data are population-based in the Hungarian Case-Control Surveillance of Congenital Abnormalities (HCCSCA) [20] thus it is possible to exclude the selection bias of the previously published hospital-based materials.
3. A special prenatal care of diabetic pregnant women was introduced in Hungary in the 1980s thus it is worth checking the efficacy of this prenatal care in the prevention of adverse birth outcomes of diabetic pregnant women.

Materials and Methods

Cases affected with different specified CAs were selected from the data set of the Hungarian Congenital Abnormality Registry (HCAR) [9] for the HCCSCA, 1980-1996. Diagnosis of CAs was based on the compulsory notification of physicians from birth until the end of the first postnatal year to the HCAR, and on autopsy reports because autopsy was mandatory for all infant deaths. Since 1984 fetal defects diagnosed in prenatal diagnostic centres with or without termination of pregnancy have also been included into the HCAR. The total (birth + fetal) prevalence of cases with CA diagnosed from the second trimester of pregnancy through the age of one year was 35 per 1000 *informative offspring* (live-born infants, stillborn fetuses and electively terminated malformed fetuses) in the HCAR, 1980-1996, and about 90% of major CAs were recorded in the HCAR during the 17 years of the study period [16].

Controls were defined as newborn infants without any CA, and they were selected the National Birth Registry of the Central Statistical Office for the HCCSCA. In most years two controls were matched to every case according to sex, birth week, and district of parents' residence.

Three Sources of Exposure Data and Confounding Factors

1. Prospective and Medically Recorded Data

Mothers were asked to send us the *prenatal maternity logbook* and other *medical records* particularly discharge summaries of their deliveries in an explanatory letter. Prenatal care was mandatory for pregnant women in Hungary, thus nearly 100% of pregnant women visited prenatal care clinics, on average 7 times during their pregnancies. The first visit was between the 6th and 12th gestational week when obstetricians recorded all pregnancy complications, maternal diseases and related drug prescriptions in the prenatal maternity logbook. The protocol of the Hungarian prenatal care includes the measurement of blood glucose level of pregnant women.

2. Retrospective Maternal Information

A structured *questionnaire,* along with a list of drugs and pregnancy supplements, diseases, plus a printed informed consent form were also mailed to the mothers immediately after the selection of cases and controls. Mothers were asked to fill in the questionnaire after the reading of list of medicinal products and diseases as memory aid and to give a signature for informed consent form.

The mean $\pm$ S.D. time elapsed between the birth or pregnancy termination and the return of the "information package" (questionnaire, logbook, etc) in our prepaid envelope was 3.5 $\pm$ 1.2 and 5.2 $\pm$ 2.9 months in the case and control groups, respectively

3. Supplementary Data Collection

Regional nurses were asked *to visit all non-respondent case mothers at home* and to help mothers to fill in the questionnaire, to evaluate available medical records and to obtain data regarding the lifestyle (smoking and drinking habits, elicit drugs during the study pregnancy) through a cross interview of mothers and their male partners or her mothers living together. Regional nurses could visit only 200 non-respondent and 600 respondent control mothers as part of two validation studies [17, 13] because the committee on ethics considered to be disturbing to visit the parents of all healthy controls. Regional nurses used the same method as in non-respondent case mothers.

The necessary information was available in 96.3% of cases (84.4% from reply to the mailing, 11.9% from the nurse visit) and in 83.0% of the controls (81.3% from reply, 1.7% from visit).

Gestational time was calculated from the first day of the last menstrual period. Beyond birth weight (g) and gestational age at delivery (wk), the rate of low birthweight (<2500 g) and large birth weight (4000 or more g) newborns, in addition the rate of preterm births (<37 weeks) and postterm birth (42 or more weeks) were analyzed on the basis of discharge summaries of inpatient obstetric clinics. The critical period of most major CAs is in the second and/or third gestational month [19].

Related *drug treatments and* use of *folic acid/multivitamin supplements* were also evaluated. Only one type of 3 mg folic acid tablet was available in Hungary during the study period. Among other *potential confounding factors,* maternal age, birth order, marital and employment status as indicators of socio-economic status [36] were evaluated.

Diagnostic Criteria of DM

Hungarian medical doctors followed the recent international consensus in the diagnosis of different types of DM.

DM was recorded in the prenatal maternity logbooks in all pregnant women in the HCCSCA, however, the type of DM was mentioned only in two-third of pregnant women. Thus the diagnosis of DM-1 was accepted on the basis of either its specified diagnosis (all pregnant women were treated with insulin) or unspecified DM with insulin treatment. The diagnosis of DM-2 was accepted on the basis of either its specified diagnosis or unspecified DM diagnosed before the conception of the study pregnancy without insulin treatment. The diagnosis of GDM was based on the recognition of DM during the study pregnancy.

We used SAS version 8.02 (SAS Institute Ins., Cary, North Carolina, USA) for statistical analyses of data.

Results

The case group included 22,843 offspring with CA, there were 79 (0.35%) pregnant women with DM-1, 77 (0.34%) pregnant women with DM-2 and 120 (0.53%) pregnant women with GDM. The numbers of livebirths was 2,146,574 in Hungary during the study period, our control sample comprised of 38,151 newborns without CA, i.e. 1.8 % of all Hungarian newborns. Of 38,151 newborns without CA, 88 (0.23%), 141 (0.37%) and 229 (0.60%) control pregnant women were affected with DM-1, DM-2 and GDM, respectively. GMD was diagnosed after the third gestational month in 92.5 % of case and 93.0% of control pregnant women. DM-1 and DM-2 were considered as chronic disease with an effect during the entire pregnancy. Of 218 pregnant women with DM-2, 6 (2.8%) while of 349 pregnant women with GDM, 62 (17.8%) were treated with insulin.

Thus, there was a higher rate of pregnant women with DM-1 in the case group as a preliminary indication of its maternal teratogenic effect.

The maternal characteristics of diabetic pregnant women showed that the mean maternal age was the highest in mothers with DM-1 (28.7 yr), and the lowest in pregnant women with DM-2 (26.0 yr) with an intermediate value in mothers with GDM (27.7 yr). All these numbers exceeded the mean age of reference sample without diabetic pregnant women (25.4 yr). The mean birth order was also somewhat higher in diabetic pregnant women. The distribution of employment status indicated a better socioeconomic status of diabetic pregnant women particularly among control mothers. The evaluation of pregnancy supplements will be mentioned later.

Among pregnancy complications, only preeclampsia-eclampsia showed a somewhat higher risk in pregnant women with DM-1.

The evaluation of other maternal diseases indicated a higher prevalence of essential hypertension in case and control pregnant women with DM-1 (16.5% and 18.2%), with DM-2 (27.3% and 22.0%) and with GDM (17.5% and 14.0%), respectively than in the reference sample (6.9%).

The use of drugs showed difference only in antidiabetic (insulin and oral antidiabetics) and antihypertensive drugs between diabetic and non-diabetic pregnant women.

Table 1 shows the birth outcomes of newborns without CA of control pregnant women with DM-1, DM-2 and GMD. (CAs may have a more drastic effect for birth outcomes than DM therefore here only the data of control newborns without CA are shown.). The mean gestational age at delivery was the same in the group of GMD and the reference sample, while DM-1 had significantly shorter, and DM-2 longer gestational age. These differences were reflected in the rate of preterm births, though it was somewhat lower in the group of GDM than in the reference sample. The mean birth weight did not follow this pattern, it was largest in the newborns of pregnant women with GDM followed by DM-1, while the mean birth weight in the group of DM-2 did not differ from the reference value. On the contrary, the largest mean birth weight in babies born to mothers with GDM, the rate of low birthweight newborns was not lower than in the reference sample. In addition the larger mean birth weight in the group of DM-1 associated with the higher (the highest) rate of low birthweight newborns in the study. The rate of postterm births was somewhat lower in the group of GDM, but the rate of large birthweight newborns was the highest. Thus these data indicate a higher risk of both small and large birthweight newborns in DM-1 and a higher risk of large birthweight newborns in the groups of GDM.

The major finding of this analysis is that the total rate of cases with CA was higher only in the group of DM-1 explained mainly by the higher risk of 4 specific types/groups of CAs had a higher risk in the offspring of mothers with DM-1. Three CA groups comprised of cases with isolated renal a/dysgenesis, obstructive CA of the urinary tract (including 2 cases with cystic dysplasia) and cardiovascular CA (including 12 cases with ventricular septal defect, but the second most common CA was transposition of the great vessels in 5 cases) while the fourth group included multiple CA. Of 9 multiple CAs, 4 (44.4%) were diagnosed as caudal dysplasia sequence

The marginal risk of diaphragmatic CAs in the offspring of mothers with DM-2 may have happened by chance because we had only 3 cases. Four multimalformed offspring of mothers with DM-2 did not fit the pattern of caudal dysplasia sequence.

In the group of pregnant women with GDM only CAs of the urinary tract showed a higher occurrence. In general, the onset of GDM occur after the third gestational months (i.e. the critical period of most major CAs), however, the critical period of some obstructive CAs of the urinary tract is in the later gestational months. Thus, this finding needs further studies to confirm or exclude this possible association. Six multimalformed offspring of mothers with GDM did not fit the pattern of caudal dysplasia sequence.

Table 1. Birth outcomes of newborn infants without CA born to mothers with DM-1, DM-2 and GDM and without DM ("none") as reference

Birth outcomes	None (N=141)		DM-1. (N=88)		DM-2. (N=141)		GDM (N=229)	
Quantitative	Mean	S.D.	Mean	S.D.	Mean	S.D.	Mean	S.D.
Gestational age, wk	39.4	2.1	38.9	2.0	39.7	1.7	39.4	1.8
Birth weight, g	3,275	510	3,324	672	3,273	438	3,390	551
Categorical	No.	%	No.	%	No.	%	No.	%
Preterm birth	3,463	9.2	11	12.5	6	4.3	16	7.0
Low birthweights	2,139	5.7	11	12.5	4	2.8	13	5.7

The total (birth + fetal) prevalences of different CAs are shown in Table 2.

Table 2. Estimation of risk for different Cas in the offspring of pregnant women with DM-1, DM-2 and GDM compared to their all matched controls

Study groups	Grand total No.	DM-1			DM-2			GDM		
		No.	%	OR 95% CI*	No.	%	OR 95% CI*	No.	%	OR 95% CI*
Controls	38,151	88	0.2	reference	141	0.4	reference	229	0.6	reference
Isolated Cas										
Neural-tube defects	1,202	3	0.2	1.1 0.3 – 3.4	5	0.4	1.1 0.5 – 2.8	7	0.6	1.0 0.5 – 2.1
Cleft lip ± palate	1,375	5	0.4	1.6 0.6 – 3.9	8	0.6	1.6 0.8 – 3.2	8	0.6	1.0 0.5 – 2.0
Cleft palate	601	3	0.5	2.2 0.7 – 6.8	1	0.2	0.4 0.1 – 3.2	1	0.2	0.3 0.0 – 2.0
Oesophageal atresia/stenosis	217	1	0.5	2.0 0.3 – 14.4	0	0.0	0.0 0.0 – 0.0	1	0.5	0.8 0.1 – 5.5
Intestinal atresia/stenosis	158	0	0.0	0.0 0.0 – 0.0	0	0.0	0.0 0.0 – 0.0	2	1.3	2.1 0.5 – 8.6
Rectal/anal atresia/stenosis	231	1	0.4	1.9 0.3 – 13.6	0	0.0	0.0 0.0 – 0.0	3	1.3	2.2 0.7 – 6.8
Renal a/dysgenesis	126	3	2.4	**10.4 3.3 – 33.5**	0	0.0	0.0 0.0 – 0.0	0	0.0	0.0 0.0 – 0.0
Obstructive urinary Cas	343	4	1.2	**5.2 1.9 – 14.3**	3	0.9	2.4 0.8 – 7.7	8	2.3	**4.0 2.0 – 8.2**
Hypospadias	3,038	7	0.2	1.0 0.5 – 2.2	9	0.3	0.8 0.4 – 1.6	14	0.5	0.8 0.4 – 1.3
Undescended testis	2,052	3	0.1	0.6 0.2 – 2.0	2	0.1	0.3 0.1 – 0.0	7	0.3	0.6 0.3 – 1.2
Exomphalos/gastroschisis	255	0	0.0	0.0 0.0 – 0.0	1	0.4	1.1 0.1 – 7.6	1	0.4	0.7 0.1 – 4.7
Hydrocephaly, congenital	314	0	0.0	0.0 0.0 – 0.0	1	0.3	0.9 0.1 – 6.2	3	1.0	1.6 0.5 – 5.0
Ear Cas	354	2	0.6	2.4 0.6 – 10.0	1	0.3	0.8 0.1 – 5.5	1	0.3	0.5 0.1 – 3.4
Cardiovascular Cas	4,480	26	0.6	**2.5 1.6 – 3.9**	16	0.4	1.0 0.6 – 1.6	28	0.6	1.0 0.7 – 1.5
Clubfoot	2,425	5	0.2	0.9 0.4 – 2.2	7	0.3	0.8 0.4 – 1.7	12	0.5	0.8 0.5 – 1.5
Limb deficiencies	548	1	0.2	0.8 0.1 – 5.7	1	0.2	0.5 0.1 – 3.5	3	0.5	0.9 0.3 – 2.8

Table 2 (Continued)

Poly/syndactyly	1,744	3	0.2	0.7 0.2 – 2.4	10	0.6	1.5 **0.8 – 2.9**	5	0.3	0.5 0.2 – 1.2
CAs of musculo-skeletal system	585	1	0.2	0.7 0.1 – 5.3	2	0.3	0.9 0.2 – 3.7	2	0.3	06 0.1 – 2.3
Diaphragmatic CAs	244	0	0.0	0.0 0.0 – 0.0	3	1.2	**3.4 1.1 – 10.6**	2	0.8	1.4 0.3 – 5.6
Other isolated CAs	1,202	2**	0.2	0.7 0.2 – 2.9	3** *	0.2	0.7 0.2 – 2.1	6** **	0.5	0.8 0.4 – 1.9
Multiple CAs	1,349	9	0.7	**2.9 1.5 – 5.8**	4	0.3	0.8 0.3 – 2.2	6	0.4	0.7 0.3 – 1.7
Total	22.843	79	0.3	**1.5 1.1 – 2.0**	77	0.3	0.9 0.7 – 1.2	120	0.5	0.9 0.7 – 1.1

*adjusted for maternal age and employment status, birth order and maternal hypertension

**congenital stenosis of trachea, congenital hiatus hernia

***cleft nose, double urethra, absent of breast

**** ankyloglossia, Hirschsprung's disease, transposition of intestine, atresia of bile duct, exstrophia of urinary bladder, congenital angulation of tibia

Finally, offspring of pregnant women with DM-I were evaluated according to folic acid supplementation. Our validation study showed that 22% of women used 1 tablet, 69% of women 2 and 9% of women consumed 3 tablets of folic acid, thus the estimated daily dose was 5.6 mg. About two-third of folic acid supplementation was based on medically recorded data on the prenatal maternity logbooks. The use of folic acid was less frequent in non-diabetic case mothers (49.3%) than in non-diabetic control mothers (64.2%). However, in general this trend was not obvious in the different types of DM in case and control mothers. Folic acid was less frequently used by case mother with DM-1 (50.5%) than in control mothers with DM-1 (54.4%), however, there was no real difference in case and control mothers with DM-2 (49.4% vs. 47.5%). On the other hand, case mothers with GDM (64.2%) used folic acid more frequently than control mothers with GDM (59.4%). The onset of folic acid supplementation was before conception in 5.1% case and 8.0% of control mothers in the total groups of DM, but these figures increased 19.0% and 23.9% in the second and 39.2% and 48.9 % in the third gestational month in case and control pregnant women, respectively. Folic acid containing micronutrient combinations, the so-called multivitamins were also evaluated, but the number of pregnant women particularly case mothers with different multivitamins was limited therefore avoided a detailed analysis. However, it is worth mentioning that folic acid containing multivitamins were not used among 79 case pregnant women with DM-1 while the occurrence of these multivitamins did not show significant difference between control mothers with or without DM-1 (6.5% vs. 8.0%).

There was no offspring with isolated neural-tube defect and renal a/dysgenesis in the folic acid supplemented subgroup, in addition there was a significant reduction in the rate of obstructive CAs of urinary tract and cleft lip± palate (Table 3). The rate of cardiovascular CAs was only somewhat lower and there was no reduction in the occurrence of multiple CAs in the subgroup of diabetic pregnant women with folic acid supplementation. Thus the total rate of CAs was not higher in the offspring of diabetic pregnant women with folic acid supplementation compared to the reference group, i.e. pregnant women without DM-1. However, the total rate of CAs was significantly higher in the offspring of diabetic pregnant women without folic acid supplementation. This preventive effect of folic acid supplementation was resulted in the critical period of the above CAs.

Table 3. Estimation of risk for different CAs in the offspring of pregnant women with or without DM-1 (as reference) and pregnant women with DM-1 with or without folic acid supplementation

Study groups	Grand total #	DM-1			Folic acid supplementation					No folic acid supplementation				
					No DM-1		DM-1			No DM-1		DM-1		
		No.	%	OR 95% CI**	No.	%	No.	%	OR (95% CI)	No.	%	No.	%	OR (95% CI)
Controls	38,151	88	0.23	reference	20,518	54.4	54	0.14	reference	17,175	45.5	34	0.09	reference
Isolated CAs														
Neural-tube defects	1,202	3	0.25	1.1 0.3 – 3.4	528	43.9	0	0.00	- (-)	674	56.1	3	0.25	2.3 (0.7 – 7.4)
Cleft lip ± palate	1,375	5	0.36	1.6 0.6 – 3.9	679	49.4	1	0.07	0.5 (0.1 – 3.3)	696	50.6	4	0.29	**2.9 (1.0 – 8.3)**
Cleft palate	601	3	0.50	2.2 0.7 – 6.8	286	47.6	1	0.17	1.0 (0.1 – 7.4)	315	52.4	2	0.33	3.3 (0-8 – 13.6)
Renal a/dysgenesis	126	3	2.38	**10.4 3.3 – 33.5**	61	48.4	0	0.00	- (-)	65	51.6	3	2.38	**24.7 (7.4 – 82.5)**
Obstructive	343	4	1.17	**5.2 1.9 – 14.3**	161	46.9	1	0.29	1.8 (0.2 – 13.0)	182	53.1	3	0.87	**8.5 (2.6 – 28.1)**
CAs of urinary tract Hypospadias	3,038	7	0.23	1.0 0.5 – 2.2	1,474	48.5	5	0.16	1.0 (0.4 – 2.6)	1,564	51.5	2	0.07	0.7 (0.2 – 2.7)
Undescended testis	2,052	3	0.15	0.6 0.2 – 2.0	1,062	51.8	2	0.10	0.6 (0.2 – 2.7)	990	48.2	1	0.05	0.5 (0.1 – 3.8)
Ear CAs	354	2	0.56	2.4 0.6 –	190	53.7	2	0.56	3.9 (0.9 –	164	46.3	0	0.00	- (-)

			10.0				16.2)					
Cardiovascular CAs	4,480	26	0.58	2.5 (1.6–3.9)	2,175	48.6	14	0.31	2.1 (1.1–3.5)	2,305	51.4	12	0.27	2.7 (1.4–5.2)
Clubfoot	2,425	5	0.21	0.9 (0.4–2.2)	1,216	50.1	3	0.12	0.8 (0.2–2.5)	1,209	49.9	2	0.08	0.8 (0.2–3.5)
Poly/syndactyly	1,744	3	0.17	0.7 (0.2–2.4)	909	52.1	1	0.06	0.4 (0.1–2.8)	835	47.9	2	0.11	1.2 (0.3–5.1)
Other isolated CAs	3,754	6*	0.16	0.7 (0.2–2.9)	1,907	50.8	3	0.08	0.5 (0-2–1.7)	1,847	49.2	3	0.08	0.8 (0.3–2.7)
Multiple CAs	1,349	9	0.67	2.9 (1.5–5.8)	631	46.8	7	0.52	3.1 (1.4–6.9)	718	53.2	2	0.15	1.4 (0.3–5.9)
Total	22,843	79	0.35	1.5 (1.1–2.0)	11,124	49.3	40	0.18	1.1 (0.7–1.7)	11,443	50.6	39	0.17	1.7 (1.1–2.7)

*congenital stenosis of trachea 1, oesophageal atresia 1, rectal stenosis 1, limb deficiency 1, congenital hiatus hernia 1, torticollis 1
**adjusted for maternal age and employment status, birth order and hypertension
Bold numbers show significant associations

Interpretation of Results

Our data confirmed the elder age and higher birth order of diabetic pregnant women [25, 32], in addition the association of DM-1 with hypertension and preeclampsia [32].

The birth outcomes are determined very much by the type of DM. The U-shaped increased risk of low and large birthweight newborns was seen in the newborns of pregnant women with DM-1. DM-2 is associated with intrauterine fetal growth delay (longer gestational age was not associated with expected larger birth weight) while GDM was associated with larger birth weight.

The major finding of our study is that the teratogenic effect of maternal DM was obvious only in the offspring of mothers with DM-1, the risk for total CAs was 1.5 fold higher. The risk of total CAs in the offspring of pregnant women with overt DM prior to conception was 4 to 8-fold higher in the previously published studies [32]. Our hope is that the lower risk figures of total CAs in the study reflects the recent progress in the specific medical care of diabetic pregnant women.

Our data confirmed the association between maternal DM-1 and caudal dysplasia sequence. Of 79 pregnant women with DM-1, 4 (5.1%) had children with caudal dysplasia sequence. Beyond this characteristic type of diabetic embryopathy, a higher rate of isolated renal a/dysgenesis, obstructive CAs of urinary tract and cardiovascular CAs, particularly transposition of great vessels was found to be associated with maternal DM-1. However, our study did not find an association of maternal DM-1 with a higher risk of neural-tube defects, congenital limb deficiencies and CA of spine in their offspring.

The latter discrepancy between the results of previous studies and our recent findings needs some discussion. On the one hand a special prenatal care was introduced for diabetic pregnant women in Hungary in the 1980s. In addition one of the important purposes of the Hungarian periconceptional service including folic acid/multivitamin supplementation introduced in 1984 was to provide a special care for diabetic pregnant women. The evaluation of about 15 thousand pregnant women showed that this service was able to prevent the maternal teratogenic effect of DM [10]. Thus these activities may contribute to the reduction of DM-1 related risk for some isolated CAs.

On the other hand the decreased rate of isolated neural-tube defects can be explained by the periconceptional high dose of folic acid [33] or folic acid-containing multivitamin supplementation [11]. In addition as our previous randomized controlled and cohort controlled trials showed periconceptional folic acid-containing multivitamin supplementation was able to reduce the occurrence of cardiovascular (particularly conotruncal) and urinary tract' (mainly obstructive) CAs as well [8, 14]. The evaluation of cases in the HCCSCA showed that the high dose of folic acid reduced the occurrence of isolated orofacial clefts [21]. However, both the results of the above two Hungarian trials [12] and the data of the HCCSCA [18] did not indicate any reduction in the rate of multiple CAs. It is worth mentioning that the use of folic acid was higher among diabetic pregnant women, particularly control mothers but the exception was just DM-1.

Thus another important message of this study is that the specific preconceptional and prenatal care of diabetic women can reduce the teratogenic risk of hyperglycemia during the critical period of CAs in pregnant women. Among this complex effect, periconceptional folic acid/multivitamin supplementation is important in the reduction of some DM-1 related CAs [2].

Finally we have to consider the chance effect that is strong in rare CAs. Two previous case-control studies found association between maternal DM and congenital limb deficiencies and CA of spine in their offspring based on 4 and 9 cases [4, 28]. Sheffield et al [40] found only one case with CA of skeleton in 410 children born to mothers with DM. Thus the explanation for the discrepancy of findings in the above and our recent studies may be the low birth prevalence of these CAs. The specific diabetic associated limb deficiency, i.e. femur or femoral head aplasia, is represented only some % in the total group of congenital limb deficiencies (0.5/1000) (15). In addition the rare CAs of spines are underrepresented in the HCAR because the lack of radiological documents in several cases.

Our study did not show a higher risk of total CAs in the offspring of pregnant women with DM-2. The teratogenic/fetotoxic risk of maternal DM depends on the severity-type [43, 31, 37], duration and efficacy of treatment [23]. Pregnant women with DM-2 in general were young with a newly onset (i.e. short duration) and not too severe DM-2 with appropriate care in our study.

GDM did also not associate with a higher risk of total CAs explained mainly with its onset after the third gestational month. However the possible association of GDM with a higher risk of obstructive CAs of urinary tract needs further studies.

We hope that the lower risk figures of total CAs (1.5-fold instead of the previous 4 to 8-fold) and the lack of higher risk of neural-tube defects and the lower risk of some other specific DM-1 related isolated CA reflect the recent progress in the specific prenatal care of diabetic pregnant women including folic acid supplementation.

The strengths of our studies are the population-based data set including 734 pregnant women with prospectively and medically recorded DM in an ethnically homogeneous Hungarian (Caucasian) population. Additional strengths are the differentiation of 3 types of DM, the matching of cases to controls without CAs; the knowledge of major potential confounders. Finally the diagnosis of medically reported CAs was checked in the HCAR and later modified, if necessary, on the basis of recent medical examination within the HCCSCA.

The major weakness of our study is that 1.2% prevalence of DM in our pregnant women indicates an underascertainment and/or undiagnosed DM particularly GDM. The diagnosis of GDM sometimes is too late or not at all, therefore these pregnant women are often treated insufficiently [38].

Our conclusions are defined according to the aims of this review

1. The differentiation of pregnant women with DM-1, DM-2, and GDM is very important because their adverse pregnancy/birth outcomes are different and obvious maternal teratogenic effect was found only in the offspring of pregnant women with DM-1.
2. The Hungarian population-based data minimized the selection bias but resulted in an underascertainment of diabetic pregnant women thus only the tip of iceberg was evaluated in the study.
3. The recent special prenatal care of diabetic pregnant women showed that the major part of maternal teratogenic effect of DM-1 is preventable with appropriate treatment of DM and folic acid supplementation.

Acknowledgments

This study was partly sponsored by a generous grant from Richter Gedeon Pharmaceuticals Ltd., Budapest, Hungary.

References

[1]   Ács N, Bánhidy F, Puho HE, Czeizel AE: Congenital abnormlities in the offspring of pregnant women with type 1, type 2 and gestational diabetes mellitus – a population-based case-control study. *Cong Anom.* (Kyoto) (submitted).

[2]   Ács N, Bánhidy F, Puho HE, Czeizel AE: Congenital abnormlities in the offspring of pregnant women with type 1 diabetes mellitus and their prevention with high dose of folic acid – a population-based case-control study. *Diabet Med.* (submitted).

[3]   Bánhidy F, Ács N, Puho HE, Czeizel AE: Comparative analysis of birth outcomes of pregnant women with type 1, type 2 and gestational diabetes mellitus – a population-based study. *Cent Eur J Med.* (submitted).

[4]   Becerra JE, Khoury MJ, Cordero JF et al. Diabetes mellitus during pregnancy and the risk for specific birth defects: A population-based case-control study. *Pediatrics,* 1990; 85: 1-9.

[5]   Ben-Haroush A, Yogev Y, Hod M: Epidemiology of gestational diabetes mellitus and its association with type 2 diabetes. *Diabet Med.* 2004; 21: 103-113.

[6]   Combs CA, Gunderson E, Kitzmiller J et al. Relationship of fetal macrosomia to maternal postprandial glucose control during pregnancy. *Diabetes Care,* 1992; 15: 1251-

[7]   Combs CA, Rosenn B, Miodovnik M et al. Sonographic EFW and macrosomia: Is there an optimum formula to predict diabetic fetal macrosomia? *J Matern Fetal Med.* 2000; 9: 55-

[8]   Czeizel AE. Reduction of urinary tract and cardiovascular defects by periconceptional multivitamin supplementation. *Am J Med Genet.* 1996; 62: 179-183.

[9]   Czeizel AE: The first 25 years of the Hungarian Congenital Abnormality Registry. *Teratology,* 1997; 55: 299-305.

[10]   Czeizel AE. Ten years experience in periconceptional care. *Eur J Obstet Gynecol Reprod Biol.* 1999; 84: 43-49.

[11]   Czeizel AE, Dudas I. Prevention of the first occurrence of neural-tube defects by periconceptional vitamin supplementation *N Engl J Med.* 1992; 327: 1832-1835.

[12] Czeizel AE, Medveczi E: No difference in the occurrence of multimalformed offspring after periconceptional multivitamin supplementation. *Obstet Gynecol.* 2003; 102: 1255-1261.

[13] Czeizel AE, Vargha P: Periconceptional folic acid/multivitamin supplementation and twin pregnancy. *Am J Obstet Gynecol.* 2004; 191: 790-794.

[14] Czeizel AE, Dobo M, Vargha P. Hungarian cohort-controlled trial of periconceptional multivitamin supplementation shows reduction in certain congenital abnormalities. *Birth Defects Res.* (Part A) 2004a;70: 853-861.

[15] Czeizel AE, Evans JA, Kodaj I, Lenz W: Congenital Limb Deficiencies in Hungary. Genetic and Teratologic Epidemiological Studies. Akadémiai Kiadó, Budapest, 1994.

[16] Czeizel AE, Intõdy Zs, Modell B: What proportion of congenital abnormalities can be prevented? *Brit Med J.* 1993; 306: 499-503.

[17] Czeizel AE, Petik D, Vargha P: Validation studies of drug exposures in pregnant women. *Pharmacoepid Drug Safety,* 2003; 12: 409-416.

[18] Czeizel AE, Puhó E, Bánhidy F: No association between periconceptional multivitamin supplementation and risk of multiple congenital abnormalities. A population-based case-control study. *Am J Med Genet Part A,* 2006; 140A 2469-2477.

[19] Czeizel AE, Puho HE, Ács N, Bánhidy F. Use of specified critical periods of different congenital abnormalities instead of the first trimester concept. *Birth Defects Res.* (Part A) 2008; 82: 139-146.

[20] Czeizel AE, Rockenbauer M, Siffel Cs, Varga E: Description and mission evaluation of the Hungarian Case-Control Surveillance of Congenital Abnormalities, 1980-1996. *Teratology,* 2001; 63:176-185.

[21] Czeizel AE, Timás L, Sárközi A: Dose-dependent effect of folic acid on the prevention of orofacial clefts. *Pediatrics,* 1999, 104: e66.

[22] Ferencz C, Rubin JN, NcCarter RJ, Clark EB. Maternal diabetes and cardiovascular Malformations: predominance of double outlet right ventricle and truncus arteriosus. *Teratology,* 1990; 41: 319-326.

[23] Greene MF. Spontaneous abortions and major malformations in women with diabetes mellitus,. *Semin Reprod Endocrinol.* 1999; 17: 127-136.

[24] Kim C, Berger DK, Chamany S: Recurrence of gestational diabetes mellitus: a systematic review. *Diabetes Care,* 2007; 30: 1314-1319.

[25] Kritz-Siverstein D, Barrett-Connor E, Wingard DL: The effect of parity on the later development of non-insulin-dependent diabetes mellitus. *N Engl J Med.* 1989; 321: 1214 -1219.

[26] Kucera J, Lenz W, Maier W: Missbildungen der Beine und der kaudalen Wirbelsaule bei Kindern diabetischer Mütter. Dtsch Med Wochenschr 1965; 90: 901-905.

[27] Loffredo CA, Wilson PD, Ferencz C. Maternal diabetes: An independent risk factors for major cardiovascular malformations with increased mortality of affected infants. *Teratology,* 2001; 64: 98-106.

[28] Martinez-Frias NL, Bemejo E, Rodriguez-Pinilla E et al. Epidemiological analysis of outcomes of pregnancy in gestational diabetic mothers. *Am J Med Genet.* 1998; 78:140-145.

[29] Meigs JB, Shader P, Sullivan LM et al. Genotype score in addition to common risk factors for prediction of type 2 diabetes. *N Engl J Med.* 2008; 359: 2208-2219.

[30] Milunsky A, Alpert E, Kitzmiller JL et al. Prenatal diagnosis of neural tube defects. The importance of serum alfa-fetoprotein in diabetic pregnant women. *Am J Obstet Gynecol.* 1982; 142: 1030-1032.

[31] Molsted-Pedersen L, Tygstrup I, Pedersen J. Congenital malformations in newborn infants of diabetic women. Correlation with maternal diabetes vascular complications. *Lancet,* 1964.1:1124-1126.

[32] Moore TR: Diabetes in pregnancy. In: Creasy RK, Resnik R, Iams JS (eds.) Maternal -Fetal Medicine. 5th ed. Saunders, Philadelphia, 2004. pp.1023-1061.

[33] MRC Vitamin Study Research Group. Prevention of neural tube defects: results of the Medical Research Council Vitamin Study. *Lancet,* 1991; 338:131-137.

[34] Nielsen GL, Norgard B, Puho E et al. Risk of specific congenital abnormalities in offspring of women with diabetes. *Diabet Med.* 2005; 22: 693-696.

[35] Passarge E, Lenz W. Syndrome of caudal regression in infants of diabetic mothers: observations of further cases. *Pediatrics,* 1966; 37: 672-675.

[36] Puho HE, Métneki J, Czeizel AE. Maternal employment status and isolated orofacial clefts in Hungary. *Cent Eur J Publ Health.* 2004; 13: 144-148.

[37] Reece EA, Sivan E, Francis G et al. Pregnancy outcomes among women with and without diabetic microvascular disease (White's classes B to FR) versus non-diabetic controls. *Am J Perinatol.* 1998; 15: 549-555.

[38] Reece EA, Leguizamón G, Wiznitzer A: Gestational diabetes: the need for a common ground. *Lancet,* 2009; 373: 1789-1797.

[39] Rusnak SL, Driscoll SG. Congenital spinal anomalies in infants of diabetic mothers. *Pediatrics,* 1965; 35: 989-995.

[40] Sheffield JS, Butler-Koster EL, Casey BM et al. Maternal diabetes mellitus and infants malformations. *Obstet Gynecol.* 202; 100: 925-930.

[41] Weigensberg MJ, Goran MI: Type 2 diabetes in children and adolescents. *Lancet,* 2009; 373:1743-1744.

[42] Weiss PAM, Coustan DR (eds.) Gestational diabetes. Springer Verlag, Wien-New York, 1988.

[43] White P. Diabetes complicating pregnancy. *Am J Obstet Gynecol.* 1937; 33: 380-385.

In: Diabetes in Women   ISBN: 978-1-61668-692-5
Editor: Eliza I. Swahn, pp. 25-45   © 2010 Nova Science Publishers, Inc.

Chapter II

Serum Levels of Insulin-Like Growth Factor-I, Pentosidine, and Adiponectin as Markers for Assessing Bone Condition in Women with Type 2 Diabetes

Ippei Kanazawa and Toru Yamaguchi[*]
Department of Internal Medicine 1, Shimane University
Faculty of Medicine, Shimane 693-8501, Japan

Abstract

Although bone mineral density (BMD) is considered as a gold standard for evaluating fracture risk in non-diabetic osteoporosis, accumulative evidence shows that patients with type 2 diabetes have high fracture rate in spite of the absence of BMD reduction, indicating that BMD is not sensitive enough to assess the risk of osteoporotic fractures

---

[*] Correspondence to: Toru Yamaguchi,
Department of Internal Medicine 1, Shimane University Faculty of Medicine,
89-1 Enya-cho, Izumo 693-8501, Japan
E-mail: yamaguch@med.shimane-u.ac.jp
Tel: +81-853-20-2183, Fax: +81-853-23-8650

in them. In addition, hyperglycemia itself is not associated with BMD or fracture risk, either. Therefore, the etiology of diabetes-related bone fragility and its diagnostic markers replacing BMD need to be explored. Advanced glycation end products (AGEs), which are produced by sequential nonenzymatic chemical glycoxidation of protein amino groups under hyperglycemia, accumulate in various tissues during normal aging, and may play a pivotal role in the development of complications including bone fragility in diabetic patients. Bone metabolism in type 2 diabetes is also affected by diabetes-related abnormality in hormonal actions of insulin and insulin-like growth factor-I (IGF-I). Our previous clinical studies have shown that serum levels of pentosidine, which is one of the well-known AGEs, as well as IGF-I could be clinically useful for assessing the risk of vertebral fractures in postmenopausal women with type 2 diabetes. On the other hand, recent animal experiments and clinical studies have indicated that osteocalcin, specifically produced by osteoblasts, acts as a hormone improving obesity and hyperglycemia, suggesting that bone metabolism and glucose/fat metabolism are etiologically related to each other. Several experiments have shown that adiponectin, one of the adipocytokines and a key mediator of visceral fat accumulation, has a stimulatory action on osteoblastogenesis and bone formation. We also found that serum adiponectin level was associated with serum osteocalcin in patients with type 2 diabetes in clinical studies. Thus, serum adiponectin may be useful for assessing not only glucose/fat metabolism but also bone metabolism including osteoblasts in diabetic patients.

Introduction

The number of patients with diabetes mellitus and osteoporosis is rapidly increasing in industrialized countries where Western-style aging societies are prevalent, and osteoporotic fractures are considered as one of major complications in elderly patients with type 2 diabetes (1). The end point of treatment for osteoporosis is the prevention of bone fractures caused by brittleness of bone. Both vertebral and hip fractures are most important osteoporotic fractures because they frequently occur and enhance the mortality of the elderly people as high as 6- to 9-fold (2,3). Therefore, it is important to assess the risk of vertebral and hip fractures in not only non-diabetic subjects but also diabetic patients.

NIH Consensus Development Panel states that bone strength primarily reflects the integration of bone density and bone quality, and BMD measurement is recommended as a gold standard for assessing bone density (4). However, no method for evaluating bone quality is clinically available at present. Neither bone formation nor resorption markers are closely related to vertebral fractures in subjects without diabetes, although bone resorption markers such as urinary collagen type I cross-linked C-telopeptide and urinary free deoxypyridinoline were significantly associated with hip fractures in several studies (5). On the other hand, the presence of vertebral fractures could be used for the assessment of bone quality in individual patients, because a large study on the incidence of vertebral fractures in postmenopausal osteoporosis showed that patients with previous vertebral fractures were more likely to suffer from new vertebral fractures (6,7) and hip fractures (6) independent of BMD than those without vertebral fractures during several-year study periods.

Accumulative evidence has indicated that BMD in patients with type 1 diabetes is lower (8-11), while that in patients with type 2 diabetes is higher than or almost the same as that in subjects without diabetes (11-14). Although patients with type 2 diabetes show no bone mass reduction, fracture risks are known to increase approximately up to 1.5-fold at the hip, proximal humerus, forearm, and foot (11,15,16). We have also shown that diabetic women have an increased risk of vertebral fractures (odds ratio 1.86) (17), while BMD values at the lumbar spine, femoral neck, or radius were not associated with the presence of vertebral fractures in them (17,18). Thus, BMD measurement is also not sensitive enough to assess the risk of vertebral fractures in diabetic women. In previous clinical studies including ours, neither bone formation nor resorption markers were associated with the presence of vertebral fractures (17,19-21), suggesting that traditional bone markers are also unable to predict vertebral fractures in diabetic patients. Since bone strength reflects the integration of bone density and bone quality, these findings suggested that patients with type 2 diabetes have poor bone quality not reflected by measurements of BMD or bone markers. Factors such as falls, visual impairment, longer diabetes duration, and insulin treatment might predispose type 2 diabetic patients to non-vertebral fractures (22). However, little is known what biochemical marker is able to evaluate diabetes-related bone fragility and to compensate for the insensitiveness of BMD or bone markers.

High glucose conditions in diabetic patients are known to impair calcium metabolism. Several studies have shown that hyperglycemia causes hypercalciuria (23), impairment of vitamin D metabolism (24), and suppresses parathyroid hormone (PTH) secretion from parathyroid (25), and resultant negative calcium balance could lead to osteopenia and bone fragility. However, a meta-analysis has revealed that hyperglycemia itself is not associated with BMD or fracture risk (11). We have also shown that HbA$_{1c}$ level was not useful for assessing the risk of vertebral fractures in patients with type 2 diabetes (18-20). Therefore, high glucose-related impairment in calcium metabolism is not likely to cause bone fragility in diabetic patients.

Advanced Glycation End Products (AGEs) and Bone Metabolism in Type 2 Diabetes

Formation of advanced glycation end products (AGEs) results from sequential nonenzymatic chemical glycoxidation of protein amino groups (26), collectively called the Maillard reaction. AGEs accumulate in various tissues including kidney, brain, and coronary artery atherosclerotic plaques during normal aging, whereas hyperglycemia results in an accelerated rate of AGE formation, suggesting that AGEs have a pivotal role in the development of complications in patients with diabetes (27,28). In addition, previous studies have revealed that AGEs accumulate in bone tissue as well (29,30), and that receptor for AGE (RAGE) is expressed in human bone-derived cells (31), suggesting that AGEs might be associated with diabetes-related bone fragility.

Several experimental studies have shown that AGEs have a negative impact on bone. AGEs inhibit the synthesis of type 1 collagen and osteocalcin as well as mature bone nodule formation in osteoblasts (32-34). We have previously demonstrated that the combination of high glucose and AGEs additionally or synergistically inhibited the mineralization of osteoblastic cells through glucose-induced increase in expression of RAGE *in vitro* (35). These findings suggest that AGEs accumulation in bone may cause osteoblastic dysfunction. AGEs are also known to increase osteoclast activity. Previous *in vitro* and *in vivo* experiments (36) have indicated that the number of resorption pits was increased when osteoclasts were cultured on AGEs-modified dentin slices, and that AGEs-bone particles were resorbed to a much greater extent than non-AGEs bone particles when implanted subcutaneously in rats. In addition, RAGE knockout mice displayed a decreased number of osteoclasts as well as a significant higher bone mass compared to wild-type mice (37).

Taken together, AGEs accumulation inhibits the differentiation and mineralization of osteoblasts, while it enhances the activity of osteoclasts, possibly leading to uncoupling bone turnover and resultant bone fragility.

AGEs accumulation in bone is also negatively associated with material properties (29,30,38). Collagen cross-links are known to play critical roles in the determination of bone strength (39). AGEs-type of cross-links, which are formed spontaneously by non-enzymatic glycation and oxidation reaction, are thought to be associated with brittleness of collagen fibers (40,41), whereas physiological cross-links (enzymatic cross-links) strengthen links of collagen fibers, and lead to the enhancement of bone strength (30,42). Spontaneously diabetic WBN/Kob rats have been reported to display a decrease in enzymatic cross-links and an increase in AGE-type of cross links despite the lack of BMD reduction, resulting in the deterioration of bone strength (43).

Among the few AGEs characterized to date, pentosidine is one of the well-known AGEs and is chemically well defined (44-46). Because the formation of pentosidine requires both glycation and oxidation, serum pentosidine levels are considered to be a useful marker for glycoxidation. Several studies have revealed that pentosidine content in cortical or trabecular bone from vertebra or femur was negatively associated with mechanical properties (29,30,38), and that pentosidine content of cortical and trabecular bone derived from patients with femoral neck fracture were higher than those of age-matched controls (47,48). However, the assessments of pentosidine content in bone are not easily done in clinical situations, because invasive procedures like bone biopsy are necessary for preparing specimens. A recent study has revealed that content of pentosidine in plasma shows a significant linear correlation with that in cortical bone (49), suggesting that serum pentosidine level could be used as a surrogate marker for its content in bone and could evaluate bone strength. We have previously shown that serum pentosidine levels were associated with prevalent vertebral fractures in postmenopausal women with type 2 diabetes (odds ratio 2.50 per SD increase) (Table 1) (20). This association is independent of BMD, suggesting that it might reflect bone quality rather than bone density. In addition, an observational cohort study has shown that urine pentosidine levels were associated with increased clinical fracture incidence in those with diabetes (relative hazard 1.42 per 1 SD increase in log pentosidine) (50). Therefore, serum and urine pentosidine levels might be useful for assessing fracture risk in women with diabetes, to which BMD or traditional bone markers are insensitive.

Table 1. Associations between the presence of vertebral fractures and serum levels of pentosidine, IGF-I and total adiponectin in female diabetic patients

	Presence of Vertebral Fractures		
Independent Variables	OR	(95% CI)	P
Pentosidine	2.50	(1.09-5.73)	0.030*
IGF-I	0.44	(0.23-0.81)	0.009*
Total Adiponectin	1.34	(0.92-1.96)	0.131

Each hormonal level was adjusted for age, body weight, body height, HbA1c, estimated GFR, duration of diabetes, duration of postmenopausal state (if female), the presence of diabetic complications, diabetes therapy, risk factors for osteoporosis, and lumbar BMD.
Unit of change; SD per increase. OR, odds ratio; CI, confidential intervals.
*;$p<0.05$

Insulin-Like Growth Factor-I (IGF-I) and Bone Metabolism in Type 2 Diabetes

Bone remodeling is regulated by systemic hormones and locally produced factors, both acting in concert to maintain bone mass (51-53). Insulin-like growth factors (IGFs) are synthesized in osteoblasts and are among the most important regulators of bone cell function due to their anabolic effects on the skeleton (54). The key role of the IGF system in the local regulation of bone formation is demonstrated by the finding that approximately 50% of basal bone cell proliferation could be blocked by inhibiting the actions of IGFs endogenously produced by bone cells in serum-free cultures (55). In osteoblast-specific knockout mice of IGF-I receptor, significant reduction in trabecular bone mass and deficient mineralization has been observed (56). On the other hand, circulating IGF-I, mainly produced in the liver via regulation by growth hormone and diet, acts in an endocrine manner, which also activates bone remodeling and exerts anabolic effects on bone tissues (57-59). Liver-specific IGF-I gene-null mice reveals a marked reduction in bone volume, periosteal circumference, and medial lateral width, suggesting that circulating levels of IGF-I also directly regulate bone growth and density (60). Indeed, our clinical studies showed that serum IGF-I levels were positively associated with BMD and inversely with the risk of vertebral fractures in postmenopausal women without diabetes (61,62). These findings suggest that serum IGF-I levels could be clinically useful for assessing bone mass and the risk of vertebral fractures in the non-diabetic population.

IGFs are thought to be linked to the pathogenesis of diabetes-related complications (63). Impaired production of IGFs could also cause bone complication in diabetes by diminishing bone cell function (54). An *in vivo* study has demonstrated that IGF-I levels in serum and cortical bone were significantly reduced in spontaneously diabetic Goto-Kakizaki rats, which displayed a significant decrease in BMD at long bone metaphyses and vertebrae (64). On the other hand, several *in vitro* studies have shown that the stimulatory actions of IGF-I on osteoblasts were blunted by high glucose concentrations or AGEs. High glucose concentrations significantly impaired the proliferative and functional responses of osteoblastic MG-63 cells to IGF-I (65). AGEs also significantly decreased IGF-I secretion in osteoblastic MC3T3-E1 cells (66). Thus, high glucose concentrations or AGEs may cause the resistance of osteoblasts to IGF-I actions in local environment.

In patients with type 2 diabetes, however, the relationship between serum IGF-I levels and bone metabolism has been little documented. We have previously indicated that serum IGF-I levels were significantly and inversely associated with the presence of vertebral fractures in postmenopausal diabetic women (odds ratio = 0.44 per SD increase) in a fashion independent of age, body statue, diabetic status, renal function, insulin secretion, or lumbar BMD (Table 1) (19). Accordingly, circulating IGF-I may have a protective effect on vertebral fractures, and this effect might be related to bone quality but not to bone density in diabetic postmenopausal women. Thus, serum IGF-I levels as well as pentosidine might be useful for assessing the risk of vertebral fractures in women with diabetes.

Adiponectin and Bone Metabolism in Type 2 Diabetes

Cumulative evidence has shown that there is a positive correlation between BMD and fat mass, suggesting that body fat and bone mass are related to each other (67-69). Several studies on adipocyte function have revealed that not only is adipose tissue an energy-storing organ but also it secretes a variety of biologically active molecules, which are named adipocytokines (70). Adiponectin is one of the adipocytokines specifically and highly expressed in visceral, subcutaneous and bone marrow fat depots (71). It is also abundantly present in plasma (72), and has been proposed to play important roles in the regulation of energy homeostasis and insulin sensitivity (73,74). Therefore, adiponectin has attracted widespread attention, especially in diabetes field, due to their beneficial anti-diabetic and anti-atherosclerotic effects.

Adiponectin is also known to be associated with bone metabolism. *In vitro* studies including ours on cultured cells have shown that adiponectin stimulates the differentiation and mineralization of osteoblasts via MAPK and AMPK signaling pathway (75-78) and induces osteoblastic differentiation of mesenchymal progenitor cells via enhancing bone morphogenetic protein-2 expression (79). In addition, it has been reported that adiponectin stimulates osteoclast differentiation via enhancing the receptor activator of nuclear factor-κB ligand (RANKL) expression and suppressing its decoy receptor, osteoprotegerin (80). These *in vitro* findings suggest that adiponectin has the ability to stimulate bone turnover by activating the differentiation of both osteoblasts and osteoclasts. On the other hand, *in vivo* animal studies present controversial results about adiponectin action on bone (77,81,82). Oshima *et al.* showed that adiponectin-overexpressing mice displayed an increase in trabecular bone mass, and that adiponectin inhibited the activity of osteoclasts and bone resorption (77). In contrast, Shinoda *et al.* found no bone abnormality in either adiponectin-deficient mice or adiponectin-overexpressing mice (81). They and Williams *et al.* showed that adiponectin had no effect on osteoclastogenesis in adiponectin-deficient mice and in RAW-264.7 cells, an osteoclastic cell line, respectively (81,82). Luo *et al.* also indicated that human osteoclast precursor cells did not have adiponectin receptors and that adiponectin had no direct effect on the differentiation of osteoclasts (80).

Clinically, several studies investigated the relationship between serum adiponectin and BMD, and controversial results were also observed. In non-diabetic women, serum adiponectin level was reported to be negatively correlated with BMD (83-85), while other studies showed no significant correlation (86-88). In diabetic patients, few studies were performed with regard to the relationship between serum adiponectin level and BMD. Lenchik *et al.* showed that after adjusting for age, gender, race, smoking, and diabetes status, serum adiponectin was inversely associated with BMD in 42 men and 38 women (86% with type 2 diabetes) (89). Tamura *et al.* showed that there was a significant positive correlation between serum adiponectin level and BMD at radius in 40 Japanese patients (28 men and 12 women) with type 2 diabetes (90). Although they investigated men and women together, some adiponectin variability is suggested to be sex-related: serum adiponectin has been reported to be higher in postmenopausal women than in men (91,92). Therefore, it would be more suitable to perform clinical studies on adiponectin after separating between men and women in order to avoid such sex-related differences. We have examined their relationship in separate genders and revealed that serum adiponectin levels were not associated with BMD or the presence of vertebral fractures in diabetic women. In contrast, the hormonal levels were significantly and negatively associated with BMD at the whole body, lumbar spine, and femoral neck, and positively with the presence of vertebral fractures in diabetic men (21). Thus, contrary to pentosidine or IGF-I, serum adiponectin level might be a useful marker for assessing the risk of vertebral fractures in men, but not in women with type 2 diabetes.

Relationships between Bone and Glucose Metabolism through the Action of Osteocalcin and Adiponectin

Several clinical studies also documented a significant positive relationship between serum adiponectin and bone markers (21,83,93,94). These findings suggest that adiponectin could also influence bone metabolism and might improve not only osteoblastic dysfunction but also low bone turnover, which is typically seen in diabetic patients and may cause bone fragility. In fact, we have previously demonstrated that serum adiponectin levels were significantly and positively correlated with serum osteocalcin levels (21,95), and that baseline serum adiponectin levels were positively correlated with changes in serum osteocalcin, undercarboxylated osteocalcin, and urinary N-terminal cross-linked telopeptide of type-I collagen during glycemic control (96). Thus, baseline serum adiponectin value could be useful for predicting augmentation in bone markers during glycemic control.

Osteocalcin, one of the osteoblast-specific proteins, has several hormonal features and is secreted in the general circulation from osteoblasts (97,98). Previous two animal studies have shown that osteocalcin derived from osteoblasts functions as a hormone regulating glucose metabolism and fat mass (99,100). Osteocalcin-knockout mice displayed decreased β-cell proliferation, glucose intolerance, and insulin sensitivity, while *ESP*-knockout mice, a model of gain of osteocalcin bioactivity, displayed increased β-cell proliferation, glucose intolerance, and insulin sensitivity (99). Moreover, osteocalcin administration regulated gene expression in β cells and adipocytes (including adiponectin expression), and suppressed the development of metabolic diseases, obesity, and type 2 diabetes in wild-type mice (100). Several clinical studies including ours have recently confirmed these experimental findings in humans. Serum osteocalcin levels are associated with serum levels of glucose and adiponectin, fat mass, as well as atherosclerosis parameters (95,101-103). We have observed that serum osteocalcin levels, but not bone-specific alkaline phosphatase, were negatively correlated with plasma glucose levels and inversely with serum adiponectin levels in postmenopausal women with type 2 diabetes (95). Kindblom *et al.* have shown that osteocalcin levels were inversely related to plasma glucose levels and fat mass in elderly non-diabetic persons (101). Fernandez-Real *et al.* have shown that serum osteocalcin levels were associated with insulin sensitivity in non-diabetes subjects (102). Pittas *et al.* have shown that serum osteocalcin levels were inversely associated with fasting plasma glucose (FPG), fasting insulin, homeostasis model assessment for insulin resistance (HOMA-IR), high-sensitivity C-reactive protein, interleukin-6, body mass index, and body fat in cross-sectional analyses (103). They also found that osteocalcin levels were associated with changes in FPG in prospective analyses (103). Taken together, these experimental and clinical findings suggest that bone metabolism and glucose metabolism are associated with each other through the action of osteocalcin and adiponectin.

Conclusion

Accumulative evidence has revealed that patients with type 2 diabetes have a higher risk of osteoporotic fractures in spite of no BMD reduction, and that BMD measurement is unable to assess fracture risk in them. Therefore, we need to explore diagnostic markers for diabetes-related bone fragility that effectively replace the insensitiveness of BMD. Previous studies have indicated that AGEs accumulation and IGF-I dysfunction were involved in diabetes-related bone fragility, and that serum levels of pentosidine and IGF-I were more potently associated with the presence of vertebral fractures than BMD or other bone turnover markers in women with type 2 diabetes. Thus, these parameters may compensate for the ineffectiveness of BMD in evaluating the risk of vertebral fractures in diabetic women. Although serum adiponectin was not useful for this purpose, its baseline value could predict augmentation in bone markers during glycemic control. It seems necessary to determine cut off values of pentosidine and IGF-I that most effectively detect incident vertebral fractures by conducting a prospective study on larger populations in near future.

References

[1]   Barrett-Connor E, Holbrook TL (1992) Sex differences in osteoporosis in older adults with non-insulin-dependent diabetes mellitus. *JAMA*, 268: 3333-3337.

[2]   Center JR, Nguyen TV, Schneider D, Sambrook PN, Eisman JA (1999) Mortality after all major types of osteoporotic fracture in men and women an observational study. *Lancet*, 353: 878-882.

[3]   Cauley JA, Thompson DE, Ensrud KC, Scott JC, Black D (2000) Risk of mortality following clinical fractures. Osteopos Int 11: 556-561.

[4]   Anonymous (2000) Osteoporosis prevention, diagnosis, and therapy. NIH Consens Statement 17: 1-45.

[5]   Looker AC, Bauer DC, Chesnut CH 3rd, Gundberg CM, Hochberg MC, Klee G, Kleerekoper M, Watts NB, Bell NH (2000) Clinical use of biochemical markers of bone remodeling: current status and future directions. *Osteoporos Int.* 11: 467-480.

[6]   Black DM, Arden NK, Palermo L, Pearson J, Cummings SR (1999) Prevalent vertebral deformities predict hip fractures and new vertebral deformities but not wrist fractures. Study of Osteoporotic Fractures Research Group. *J Bone Miner Res.* 14: 821-828.

[7]   Liberman UA, Weiss SR, Broll J, Minne HW, Quan H, Bell NH, Rodriguez-Portales J, Downs RW Jr, Dequeker J, Favus M (1995) Effect of oral adendronate on bone mineral density and the incidence of fractures in postmenopausal osteoporosis. The Alendronate Phase III Osteoporosis Treatment Study Group. *N Engl J Med.* 333: 1437-1443.

[8]   Hampson G, Evans C, Petitt RJ, Evans WD, Eoodhead SJ, Peters JR, Ralston SH (1998) Bone mineral density, collagen type 1 alpha 1 genotypes and bone turnover in postmenopausal women with diabetes mellitus. *Diabetologia*, 41: 1314-1320.

[9]   Munoz-Torres M, Jodar E, Escobar-Jimenez F, Lopez-Ibarra PJ, Luna JD (1996) Bone mineral density measured by dual X-ray absorptiometry in Spanish patients with insulin-dependent diabetes mellitus. Calcif Tissue Int 58: 316-319.

[10]   Jehle PM, Jehle DR, Mohan S, Bohm BO (1998) Serum levels of insulin-like growth factor system components and relationship to bone metabolism in type 1 and type 2 diabetes mellitus patients. *J Endocrinol.* 159: 297-306.

[11]   Vestergaard P (2007) Discrepancies in bone mineral density and fracture risk in patients with type 1 and type 2 diabetes –a meta-analysis. *Osteoporos Int.* 18: 427-444.

[12]   van Daele PL, Stolk RP, Berger H, Algra D, Grobbee DE, Hofman A, Birkenhager JC, Pols HA (1995) Bone density in non-insulin-dependent diabetes mellitus. The Rotterdam Study. *Am Intern Med.* 122: 409-414.

[13]   Isaia GC, Ardissone P, Di Stefano M, Ferrari D, Martina V, Porta M, Tagliabue M, Molinatti GM (1999) Bone metabolism in type 2 diabetes mellitus. *Acta Diabetol.* 36: 35-38.

[14]   Schwartz AV, Sellmeyer DE, Ensrud KE, Cauley JA, Tabor HK, Schreiner PJ, Jamal SA, Black DM, Cummings SR (2001) Older women with diabetes have an increased risk of fracture: a prospective study. *Journal of Clinical Endocrinology and Metabolism*, 86: 32-38.

[15]   Lipscombe LL, Jamal SA, Booth GL, Hawker GA (2007) The risk of hip fractures in older individuals with diabetes: a population-based study. Diabetes Care 30: 835-841.

[16]   Strotmeyer ES, Cauley JA, Schwartz AV, Nevitt MC, Resnick HE, Bauer DC, Tylavsky FA, de Rekeneire N, Harris TB, Newman AB (2005) Nontraumatic fracture risk with diabetes mellitus and impaired fasting glucose in older white and black adults: the health, aging, and body composition study. Arch of Intern Med 165: 1612-1617.

[17]   Yamamoto M, Yamaguchi T, Yamauchi M, Kaji H, Sugimoto T (2009) Diabetic patients have an increased risk of vertebral fractures independent of bone mineral density or diabetic complications. *J Bone Miner Res.* 24: 702-709.

[18] Yamamoto M, Yamaguchi T, Yamauchi M, Kaji H, Sugimoto T (2007) Bone mineral density is not sensitive enough to assess the risk of vertebral fractures in type 2 diabetic women. *Calcif Tissue Int.* 80: 353-358.

[19] Kanazawa I, Yamaguchi T, Yamamoto M, Yamauchi M, Yano S, Sugimoto T (2007) Serum insulin-like growth factor-I is associated with the presence of vertebral fractures in postmonopausal women with type 2 diabetes mellitus. *Osteoporos Int.* 18: 1675-1681.

[20] Yamamoto M, Yamaguchi T, Yamauchi M, Yano S, Sugimoto T (2008) Serum pentosidine levels are positively associated with the presence of vertebral fractures in postmenopausal women with type 2 diabetes. *J Clin Endocrinol Metab.* 93: 1013-1019.

[21] Kanazawa I, Yamaguchi T, Yamamoto M, Yamauchi M, Yano S, Sugimoto T (2009) Relationships between serum adiponectin levels versus bone mineral density, bone metabolic markers, and vertebral fractures in type 2 diabetes mellitus. *Eur J Endocrinol.* 160: 265-273.

[22] Ivers RQ, Cumming RG, Mitchell P, Peduto AJ (2001) Blue Mountains Eye Study: Diabetes and risk of fracture: The Blue Mountains Eye Study. *Diabetes Care,* 24: 1198-1203.

[23] Raskin P, Stevenson MR, Barilla DE, Pak CY (1978) The hypercalciuria of diabetes mellitus: its amelioration with insulin. *Clin Endocrinol.* (Oxf) 9: 329-335.

[24] Ishida H, Cunningham NS, Henry HL, Norman AW (1988) The number of 1,25-dihydroxyvitamin D3 receptors is decreased in both intestine and kidney of genetically diabetic db/db mice. *Endocrinology,* 122: 2436-2443.

[25] Sugimoto T, Ritter C, Morrissey J, Hayes C, Statopolsky E (1990) Effects of high concentrations of glucose on PTH secretion in parathyroid cells. *Kidney Int.* 37: 1522-1527.

[26] Brownlee M (1995) Advanced protein glycosylation in diabetes and aging. *Annu Rev Med.* 46: 223-234.

[27] Brownlee M, Cerami A, Vlassara H (1988) Advanced glycosylation end products in tissue and the biochemical basis of diabetic complications. *N Engl J Med.* 318: 1315-1321.

[28] Goldin A, Beckman JA, Schmidt AM, Creager MA (2006) Advanced glycation end products sparking the development of diabetic vascular injury. *Circulation,* 114: 597-605.

[29] Hernandez CJ, Tang SY, Baumbach BM, Hwu PB, Sakkee AN, van der Ham F, DeGroot J, Bank RA, Keaveny TM (2005) Trabecular microfracture and the influence of pyridinium and non-enzymatic glycation-mediated collagen cross-links. *Bone*, 37: 825-832.

[30] Wang X, Shen X, Li X, Agrawal CM (2002) Age-related changes in the collagen network and toughness of bone. *Bone*, 31: 1-7.

[31] Takagi M, Kasayama S, Yamamoto T, Motomura T, Hashimoto K, Yamamoto H, Sato B, Okada S, Kishimoto T (1997) Advanced glycation end-products stimulate interleukin-6 production by human bone-derived cells. *J Bone Miner Res.* 12: 439-446.

[32] Yamamoto T, Ozono K, Miyauchi A, Kasayama S, Kojima Y, Shima M, Okada S (2001) Role of advanced glycation end products in adynamic bone disease in patients with diabetic nephropathy. *Am J Kidney Dis.* 38: S161-S164.

[33] Katayama Y, Akatsu T, Yamamoto M, Kugai N, Nagata N (1996) Role of nonenzymatic glycosylation of type 1 collagen in diabetic osteopenia. *J Bone Miner Res.* 11: 931-937.

[34] Sanguineti R, Storace D, Monacelli F, Federici A, Odetti P (2008) Pentosidine effects on human osteoblasts in vitro. *Ann N Y Acad Sci.* 1126: 166-172.

[35] Ogawa N, Yamaguchi T, Yano S, Yamauchi M, Yamamoto M, Sugimoto T (2007) The combination of high glucose and advanced glycation end-products (AGEs) inhibits the mineralization of osteoblastic MC3T3-E1 cells through glucose-induced increase in the receptor for AGEs. *Horm Metab Res.* 39: 871-875.

[36] Miyata T, Notoya K, Yoshida K, Horie K, Maeda K, Kurokawa K, Taketomi S (1997) Advanced glycation end products enhance osteoclast-induced bone resorption in cultured mouse unfractionated bone cells and in rats implanted subcutaneously with devitalized bone particles. *J Am Soc Nephrol.* 8: 260-270.

[37] Ding KH, Wang ZZ, Hamrick MW, Deng ZB, Zhou L, Kang B, Yan SL, She JX, Stern DM, Isales CM, Mi QS (2006) Disordered osteoclast formation in RAGE-deficient mouse establishes an essential role for RAGE in diabetes related bone loss. *Biochem Biophys Res Commun.* 340: 1091-1097.

[38] Viguet-Carrin S, Roux JP, Arlot ME, Merabet Z, Leeming DJ, Byrjalsen I, Delmas PD, Bouxsein ML (2006) Contribution of the advanced glycation end product pentosidine and of maturation of type I collagen

to compressive biomechanical properties of human lumbar vertebrae. Bone 39: 1073-1079.

[39] Saito M, Marumo K. Collagen cross-links as a determinant of bone quality: a possible explanation for bone fragility in aging, osteoporosis, and diabetes mellitus. Osteoporos Int, Epub ahead of print.

[40] Garnero P, Borel O, Gineyts E, Duboeuf F, Solberg H, Bouxsein ML, Christiansen C, Delmas PD (2006) Extracellular post-translational modifications of collagen are major determinants of biomechanical properties of fetal bovine cortical bone. Bone 38: 300-309.

[41] Vashishth D (2007) The role of the collagen matrix in skeletal fragility. *Curr Osteoporos Rep.* 5: 62-66.

[42] Banse X, Sims TJ, Bailey AJ (2002) Mechanical properties of adult vertebral cancellous bone: correlation with collagen intermolecular cross-links. J Bone Miner Res 17: 1621-1628.

[43] Saito M, Fujii K, Mori Y, Marumo K (2006) Role of collagen enzymatic and glycation induced cross-links as a determinant of bone quality in spontaneously diabetic WBN/Kob rats. *Osteoporos Int.* 17: 1514-1523.

[44] Odetti P, Fogarty J, Sell DR, Monnier VM (1992) Chromatographic quantitation of plasma and erythrocyte pentosidine in diabetic and uremic subjects. *Diabetes,* 41: 153-159.

[45] Monnier VM, Sell DR, Nagaraj RH, Miyata S, Grandhee S, Odetti P, Ibrahim SA (1992) Maillard reaction-mediated molecular damage to extracellular matrix and other tissue proteins in diabetes, aging, and uremia. *Diabetes,* 41: 36-41.

[46] Grandhee SK, Monnier VM (1991) Mechanism of formation of the Maillard protein cross-link pentosidine. Glucose, fructose, and ascorbate as pentosidine precursors. *J Biol Chem.* 266: 11649-11653.

[47] Saito M, Fujii K, Soshi S, Tanaka T (2006) Reductions in degree of mineralization and enzymatic collagen cross-links and increases in glycation-induced pentosidine in the femoral neck cortex in cases of femoral neck fracture. *Osteoporos Int.* 17: 986-995.

[48] Saito M, Fujii K, Marumo K (2006) Degree of mineralization-related collagen crosslingking in the femoral neck cancellous bone in cases of hip fracture and controls. Calcif Tissue Int 79: 160-168.

[49] Odetti P, Rossi S, Monacelli F, Poggi A, Cirnigliaro M, Federici M, Federici A (2005) Advanced glycation end products and bone loss during aging. *Ann N Y Acad Sci.* 1043: 710-717.

[50] Schwartz AV, Garnero P, Hillier TA, Sellmeyer DE, Strotmeyer ES, Feingold KR, Resnick HE, Tylavsky FA, Black DM, Cummings SR, Harris TB, Bauer DC; for the Health, Aging, and Body Composition Study (2009) Pentosidine and increased fracture risk in older adults with type 2 diabetes. *J Clin Endocrinol Metab.* 94: 2380-2386.

[51] Canalis E (1983) The hormonal and local regulation of bone formation. Endocr Rev 4: 62-77.

[52] Mohan S, Baylink DJ (1991) Bone growth factors. *Clin Orthop Relat Res.* 263: 30-48.

[53] Ueland T (2004) Bone metabolism in relation to alterations in systemic growth hormone. Growth Horm IGF Res 14: 404-417.

[54] McCarthy TL, Centrella M, Canalis E (1989) Insulin-like growth factor (IGF) and bone. Connect Tissue Res 20: 277-282.

[55] Mohan S (1993) Insulin-like growth factor binding proteins in bone cell regulation. *Growth Regul.* 3: 67-70.

[56] Zhang M, Xuan S, Bouxsein ML, von Stechow D, Akeno N, Faugere MC, Malluche H, Zhao G, Rosen CJ, Efstratiadis A, Clemens TL (2002) Osteoblast-specific knockout of the insulin-like growth factor (IGF) receptor gene reveals and essential role of IGF signaling in bone matrix mineralization. *J Biol Chem.* 277: 44005-44012.

[57] Johansson AG, Lindh E, Ljunghall S (1992) Insulin-like growth factor I stimulates bone turnover in osteoporosis. Lancet 339: 1619.

[58] Schwander JC, Hauri C, Zapf J, Froesch ER (1983) Synthesis and secretion of insulin-like growth factor and its binding protein by the perfused rat liver: dependence on growth hormone status. *Endocrinology,* 113: 297-305.

[59] Spencer EM, Liu CC, Si EC, Howard GA (1991) In vivo actions of insulin-like growth factor-I (IGF-I) on bone formation and resorption in rats. *Bone,* 12: 21-26.

[60] Yakar S, Rosen CJ, Beamer WG, Ackert-Bicknell CL, Wu Y, Liu JL, Ooi GT, Setser J, Frystyk J, Boisclair YR, LeRoith D (2002) Circulating levels of IGF-I directly regulate bone growth and density. *J Clin Invest.* 110: 771-781.

[61] Sugimoto T, Nishiyama K, Kuribayashi F, Chihara K (1997) Serum levels of insulin-like growth factor (IGF) I, IGF-binding protein (IGFBP)-2, and IGFBP-3 in osteoporotic patients with and without spinal fractures. *J Bone Miner Res.* 12 1272-1279.

[62] Yamaguchi T, Kanatani M, Yamauchi M, Kaji H, Sugishita T, Baylink DJ, Mohan S, Chihara K, Sugimoto T (2006) Serum levels of insulin-like growth factor (IGF); IGF-binding proteins-3, -4, and -5; and their relationships to bone mineral density and the risk of vertebral fractures in postmenopausal women. Calcif Tissue Int 78: 18-24.

[63] Thrailkill KM (2000) Insulin-like growth factor-I in diabetes mellitus: its physiology, metabolic effects, and potential clinical utility. *Diabetes Technol Ther*. 2: 69-80.

[64] Ahmad T, Ugarph-Morawski A, Lewitt MS, Li J, Saaf M, Brismar K (2008) Diabetic osteopathy and the IGF system in the Goto-Kakizaki rat. *Growth Horm IGF Res*. 18: 404-411.

[65] Terada M, Inaba M, Yano Y, Hasuma Y, Nishizawa Y, Morii H, Otani S (1998) Growth-inhibitory effect of a high glucose concentration on osteoblast-like cells. *Bone,* 22: 17-23.

[66] McCarthy AD, Etcheverry SB, Cortizo AM (2001) Effect of advanced glycation endproducts on the secretion of insulin-like growth factor-I and its binding proteins: role in osteoblast development. Acta Diabetol 38: 113-122.

[67] Lim S, Joung H, Shin CS, Lee HK, Kim KS, Shin EK, Kim HY, Lim MK, Cho SI (2004) Body composition changes with age have gender-specific impacts on bone mineral density. *Bone,* 35: 792-798.

[68] Felson DT, Zhang Y, Hannan MT, Anderson JJ (1993) Effects of weight, and body mass index on bone mineral density in men and women. J Bone Miner Res 8: 567-573.

[69] Glauber HS, Vollmer WM, Nevitt MC, Ensrud KE, Orwoll ES (1995) Body weight versus body fat distribution, adiposity, and frame size as predictors of bone density. *J Clin Endocrinol Metab*. 80: 1118-1123.

[70] Maeda K, Okubo K, Shimomura I, Mizuno K, Matsuzawa Y, Matsubara K (1997) Analysis of an expression profile of genes in the human adipose tissue. *Gene,* 190: 227-235.

[71] Weyer C, Funahashi T, Tanaka S, Hotta K, Matsuzawa Y, Pratley RE, Tataranni PA (2001) Hypoadiponectemia in obesity and type 2 diabetes: close association with insulin resistance and hyperinsulinemia. *J Clin Endocrinol Metab*. 86: 1930-1935.

[72] Arita Y, Kihara S, Ouchi N, Takahashi M, Maeda K, Miyagawa J, Hotta K, Shimomura I, Nakamura T, Miyaoka K, Kuriyama H, Nishida M, Yamashita S, Okubo K, Matsubara K, Muraguchi M, Ohmoto Y, Funahashi T, Matsuzawa Y (1999) Paradoxical decrease of an adipose-

specific protein, adiponectin, in obesity. *Biochem Biophys Res Commun.* 257: 79-83.

[73] Combs TP, Berg AH, Obici S, Scherer PE, Rossetti L (2001) Endogenous glucose production is inhibited by the adipose-derived protein Acrp30. *J Clin Invest.* 108: 1875-1881.

[74] Berg AH, Combs TP, Du X, Brownlee M, Scherer PE (2001) The adipocyte-secreted protein Acrp30 enhances hepatic insulin action. Nature Med 7: 947-953.

[75] Kanazawa I, Yamaguchi T, Yano S, Yamauchi M, Yamamoto M, Sugimoto T (2007) Adiponectin and AMP kinase activator stimulate proliferation, differentiation, and mineralization of osteoblastic MC3T3-E1 cells. BMC Cell Biol 8: 51.

[76] Berner HS, Lyngstadaas SP, Spahr A, Monjo M, Thommesen L, Drevon CA, Syversen U, Reseland JE (2004) Adiponectin and its receptors are expressed in bone-forming cells. *Bone*, 35: 842-849.

[77] Oshima K, Nampei A, Matsuda M, Iwaki M, Fukuhara A, Hashimoto J, Yoshikawa H, Shimomura I (2005) Adiponectin increases bone mass by suppressing osteoclast and activating osteoblast. *Biochem Biophys Res Commun.* 331: 520-526.

[78] Luo XH, Guo LJ, Yuan LQ, Xie H, Zhou HD, Wu XP, Liao EY (2005) Adiponectin stimulates human osteoblasts proliferation and differentiation via the MAPK signaling pathway. *Exp Cell Res.* 309: 99-109.

[79] Lee HW, Kim SY, Kim AY, Lee EJ, Choi JY, Kim JB (2009) Adiponectin stimulates osteoblast differentiation through induction of COX2 in mesenchymal progenitor cells. *Stem Cells*, 27: 2254-2262.

[80] Luo XH, Guo LJ, Xie H, Yuan LQ, Wu XP, Zhou HD, Liao EY (2006) Adiponectin stimulates RANKL and inhibits OPG expression in human osteoblasts through the MAPK signaling pathway. J Bone Miner Res 21: 1648-1656.

[81] Shinoda Y, Yamaguchi M, Ogata N, Akune T, Kubota N, Yamauchi T, Terauchi Y, Kadowaki T, Takeuchi Y, Fukumoto S, Ikeda T, Hoshi K, Chung U, Nakamura K, Kawaguchi H (2006) Regulation of bone formation by adiponectin through autocrine/paracrine and endocrine pathways. *J Cell Biochem.* 99: 196-208.

[82] Williams GA, Wang Y, Callon KE, Watson M, Lin JM, Lam JB, Costa JL, Orpe A, Broom N, Naot D, Reid IR, Cornish J (2009) In vivo and in vitro effects of adiponectin on bone. *Endocrinology*, 150: 3603-3610.

[83] Richards JB, Valdes AM, Burling K, Perks UC, Spector TD (2007) Serum adiponectin and bone mineral density in women. *J Clin Endocrinol Metab.* 92: 1517-1523.

[84] Jürimäe J, Jürimäe T (2007) Adiponectin is a predictor of bone mineral density in middle-aged premenopausal women. *Osteoporos Int.* 18: 1253-1259.

[85] Jürimäe J, Rembel K, Jürimäe T, Rehand M (2005) Adiponectin is associated with bone mineral density in perimenopausal women. *Horm Metab Res.* 37: 297-302.

[86] Kontogianni M, Dafni UG, Routsias J, Skopouli FN (2004) Blood leptin and adiponectin as possible mediators of the relation between fat mass and BMD in perimenopausal women. *J Bone Miner Res.* 19: 546-551.

[87] Huang KC, Cheng WC, Yen RF, Tsai KS, Tai TY, Yang WS (2004) Lack of independent relationship between plasma adiponectin, leptin levels and bone density in nondiabetic female adolescents. *Clin Endocrinol.* 61: 204-208.

[88] Jürimäe J, Jürimäe T (2007) Plasma adiponectin concentration in healty pre- and postmenopausal women: relationship with body composition, bone mineral, and metabolic cariables. *Am J Physiol Endocrinol Metab.* 293: E42-47.

[89] Lenchik L, Register TC, Hsu FC, Lohman K, Nicklas BJ, Freedman BI, Langefeld CD, Carr JJ, Bowden DW (2003) Adiponectin as a novel determinant of bone mineral density and visceral fat. Bone 33: 646-651.

[90] Tamura T, Yoneda M, Yamane K, Nakanishi S, Nakashima R, Okubo M, Kohno N (2007) Serum leptin and adiponectin are positively associated with bone mineral density at the distal radius in patients with type 2 diabetes mellitus. *Metabolism,* 56: 623-628.

[91] Pajvani UB, Hawkins M, Combs TP, Rajala MW, Doebber T, Berger JP, Wagner JA, Wu M, Knopps A, Xiang AH, Utzschneider KM, Kahn SE, Olefsky JM, Buchanan TA, Scherer PE (2004) Complex distribution, not absolute amount of adiponectin, correlates with thiazolidinedione-mediated improvement in insulin sensitivity. *J Biol Chem.* 279: 12152-12162.

[92] Waki H, Yamauchi T, Kamon J, Ito Y, Uchida S, Kita S, Hara K, Hada Y, Vasseur F, Froguel P, Kimura S, Nagai R, Kadowaki T (2003) Impaired multimerization of human adiponectin mutants associated with diabetes: molecular structure and multimer formation of adiponectin. *J Biol Chem.* 278: 40352-40363.

[93] Peng XD, Xie H, Zhao Q, Wu XP, Sun ZQ, Liao EY (2008) Relationships between serum adiponectin, leptin, resistin, visfatin levels and bone mineral density, and bone biochemical markers in Chinese men. *Clinica Chimica Acta,* 387: 31-35.

[94] Gregorio F, Cristallini S, Stanteusanio F, Filipponi P, Fumelli P (1994) Osteopenia associated with non-insulin-dependent diabetes mellitus: what are the causes? *Diabetes Res Clin Pract.* 23: 43-54.

[95] Kanazawa I, Yamaguchi T, Yamamoto M, Yamauchi M, Kurioka S, Yano S, Sugimoto T (2009) Serum osteocalcin level is associated with glucose metabolism and atherosclerosis parameters in type 2 diabetes mellitus. *J Clin Endocrinol Metab.* 94: 45-49.

[96] Kanazawa I, Yamaguchi T, Yamauchi M, Yamamoto M, Kurioka S, Yano S, Sugimoto T (2009) Adiponectin is Associated with Changes in Bone Markers during Glycemic Control in Type 2 Diabetes Mellitus. *J Clin Endocrinol Metab.* 94: 3031-3037.

[97] Hauschka PV, Lian JB, Cole DE, Gundberg CM (1989) Osteocalcin and matrix protein: vitamin K-dependent proteins in bone. *Physiol Rev.* 69: 990-1047.

[98] Price PA (1989) Gla-containing proteins of bone. *Connect Tissue Res.* 21:51-57.

[99] Lee NK, Sowa H, Hinoi E, Ferron M, Ahn JD, Confavreux C, Dacquin R, Mee PJ, McKee MD, Jung DY, Zhang Z, Kim JK, Mauvais-Jarvis F, Ducy P, Karsenty G (2007) Endocrine regulation of energy metabolism by the skeleton. *Cell,* 130: 456-469.

[100] Ferron M, Hinoi E, Karsenty G, Ducy P (2008) Osteocalcin differentially regulates beta cell and adipocyte gene expression and affects the development of metabolic diseases in wild-type mice. *Proc Natl Acad Sci USA*, 105: 5266-5270.

[101] Kindblom JM, Ohlsson C, Ljunggren O, Karlsson MK, Tivesten A, Smith U, Mellstrom D (2009) Plasma osteocalcin is inversely related to fat mass and plasma glucose in elderly Swedish men. *J Bone Miner Res.* 24: 785-791.

[102] Fernandez-Real JM, Izquierdo M, Ortega F, Gorostiaga E, Gomez-Ambrosi J, Moreno-Navarrete JM, Fruhbeck G, Martinez C, Idoate F, Salvador J, Forga L, Ricart W, Ibanez J (2009) The relationship of serum osteocalcin concentration to insulin secretion, sensitivity, and disposal with hypocaloric diet and resistance training. *J Clin Endocrinol Metab.* 94: 237-245.

[103] Pitass AG, Harris SS, Eliades M, Stark P, Dawson-Hughes B (2009) Association between serum osteocalcin and markers of metabolic phenotype. *J Clin Endocrinol Metab.* 94: 827-832.

In: Diabetes in Women   ISBN: 978-1-61668-692-5
Editor: Eliza I. Swahn, pp. 47-65   © 2010 Nova Science Publishers, Inc.

Chapter III

Women's Knowledge and Self-Management of Diabetes

Julie E. Byles [*], *Anne F. Young, and Julia M. Lowe*
Research Centre for Gender, Health and Ageing,
The University of Newcastle, Australia

Abstract

Self management of diabetes is an essential component of diabetes
care, and to achieve good self-care people with diabetes should be
knowledgeable about the purpose and clinical utility of diagnostic tests
and monitoring. In this study we sought to identify and describe women's
attitudes to diabetes, their knowledge of diabetes, their self management
behaviours, and their health outcomes and, to explore the
interrelationship between these factors. The study involved analysis of

---

[*] Author for correspondence:
Julie Byles
Research Centre for Gender and Health
University of Newcastle
Callaghan NSW 2308
AUSTRALIA
Phone: +61 2 49138643
Fax: +61 2 49138321
Email: julie.byles@newcastle.edu.au

survey data from 223 women aged 50-55 years, and 655 women aged 75-80 years participating in the Australian Longitudinal Study on Women's Health, who reported having diabetes. Survey data included socio-demographic and health variables, type and duration of diabetes, level and frequency of diabetes care, knowledge, attitudes and self-care practices, and access to diabetes-related health services and diabetes education services. Most women expressed positive attitudes regarding their adjustment to having diabetes although a large proportion of women did not engage in appropriate behaviours and preventive activities. In general the women in both age groups had less than optimal levels of knowledge, although women who had attended a diabetes education centre had better knowledge scores. Better knowledge was correlated with better behaviours (in both age groups) and with better health outcomes (among older women). The results of the study indicate that, at a community level, there is a great need to improve knowledge and behaviours among the growing population of women with diabetes, particularly those with Type II diabetes and older people. The results also provide strong support for the work of diabetes education centres.

Introduction

The cornerstones of good diabetes care are considered to be education, multidisciplinary care and good self-management (Diabetes Australia and RACGP 2005; Funnell and Anderson 2004). Numerous studies have shown that patient education and self-management programs can reduce costs and enhance quality of life for people with diabetes (e.g. Tomky 1999; Fleming et al. 2001; Oosthuizen et al. 2002; Deakin et al. 2005; Salas et al. 2009). However, self-management can be complex and involves close day-to-day monitoring of the condition and maintenance of self-care behaviours (Corser 2009). People with diabetes must make frequent changes to medications, diet, physical activity, and other lifestyle factors (Seley and Weinger 2007). Self-management also requires that people with diabetes are knowledgeable about their condition, and its treatment and monitoring. In particular, patients should be knowledgeable about the purpose and clinical utility of diagnostic tests and monitoring, and awareness of test results has been found to be significantly associated both with actual HbA1c control and with receiving recommended diabetes services (Setter et al 2003; Heisler et al. 2003). However, studies indicate that many people with diabetes have poor knowledge of diabetes tests and monitoring (Jorgensen, Polivka and Lennie 2002), and are therefore particularly vulnerable to poorer health outcomes (Nasmith et al. 2004; Peyrot et al. 2006; Nagelkerk, Reick and Meengs 2006; Keers et al 2006).

Studies also show that people with diabetes do not receive all elements of optimal care (Beckles eta al. 1998; Saaddine et al. 2002; Peyrot et al. 2006; Giugliano et al. 2009). According to data from the United States National Health and Nutrition Examination Survey (NHANES III – collected during 1988–1995), a substantial gap exists between recommended diabetes care and the care patients actually receive. Among the NHANES III participants, 18% had poor glycemic control reflected by hemoglobin A1c (HBA1c) level > 9.5%, 34% had high blood pressure, and 58% had elevated cholesterol levels. During the year preceding the survey, 63% had a dilated eye examination and 55% had a foot examination (Saaddine et al. 2002). A more recent assessment of diabetes care in the United States suggests that diabetes care and intermediate outcomes have improved since the NHANES III data were collected. However, there are still important opportunities for further improvement (Saaddine et al. 2006).

While studies of clinic populations indicate room for improvement in diabetes knowledge and self-management practices, they are likely to underestimate the true need for diabetes education at a community level. The impact of diabetes education at a population level is likely to be affected by a number of factors. These include not only the severity and duration of the person's condition but also their personal characteristics and social context. For example, patients who are more effective and confident in self-management may also be more effective in securing necessary diabetes services – they may be more informed about the services they need, may remind providers, or follow through and have ordered tests (Heisler 2003; Corser 2009). Social support is another factor that may influence whether people access education and their adherence with health care advice.

An understanding of the availability and effectiveness of the health care received by people with diabetes at a community level requires a large body of data collected from a representative sample of people of varying socioeconomic circumstances. The Australian Longitudinal Study on Women's Health (ALSWH) provides an important opportunity to gain insights into the factors affecting the health and well being of women with diabetes. The ALSWH aims to examine the relationships between biological, psychological, social and lifestyle factors and women's physical health, emotional well being and use of health care services. The 20-year study began in 1996 with a national random sample of more than 40,000 community dwelling women (Brown et al. 1998). The prevalence of diabetes among these women, factors associated with diabetes and their health and use of health care services has been reported earlier (Young et al 2005).

This earlier analysis included 12,328 women born in 1946-1951, and 10,421 women born 1921-1926 who had completed our baseline and first follow up surveys (Survey 1 and Survey 2). Among the women in the 1946-51 cohort, 236 women (1.9%) reported being diagnosed with diabetes prior to 1996 (Survey 1), and 141 women (1.1%) were diagnosed between 1996 and 1998 (Survey 2). Of the women in the 1921-26 cohort, 840 women (8.1%) had been diagnosed with diabetes prior to 1996 and 266 new cases (2.6%) were diagnosed between 1996 and 1999 (Survey 2 for these older women). Compared to other women in these cohorts, women with diabetes tended to have lower education and, among the mid-age women, were less likely to be employed in paid work and more likely to be of Indigenous origin. Women with diabetes were also much more likely to have hypertension, heart disease and eyesight problems and the prevalence of these conditions was much greater among older women than among mid-age women. There were striking differences in body mass index between women with and without diabetes. Of the mid-age women who were diagnosed with diabetes between the first and second surveys, 80% were overweight at Survey 1, with one-quarter having BMI greater than 35. Less than half the women in this study had adequate levels of physical activity. Among mid-age women, those diagnosed with diabetes between Survey 1 and Survey 2 were least likely to be doing adequate exercise; among the older women those diagnosed with diabetes at any time were least likely to be doing adequate exercise. The majority of women were non-smokers and only a small proportion drank alcohol at levels considered to be harmful to health. At Survey 1, one-quarter of the mid-age women and half the older women with diabetes were taking four or more prescribed medications daily. This percentage increased over the period between Survey 1 and Survey 2, with high rates of polypharmacy among women with diabetes (Young et al 2005).

In this earlier research we also assessed the quality of care received by women reporting diabetes. This was done by linking the survey data to data from Medicare Australia, the universal health insurer for all people in Australia. These data showed that Use of HbA1c tests was less than the recommended 6-12 monthly, with less than 60% of the women with diabetes having a record of this test in each year from 1997 to 2002. However, there was a trend over the five-year period for a greater percentage of women with diabetes to have the test at least once a year. Rates of testing microalbuminuria were low, rising from about 10% in 1997 to 20% in 2001. Similarly, rates of lipids testing increased over the five-year period but were far from conforming to the best practice guidelines of at least annual testing (Young et al 2005).

In this further study, we examine the individual characteristics of the women in the study who manage their diabetes well, in the context of their social circumstances. This research seeks to explore the interrelationship between the many factors that lead to variability in health outcomes for women with diabetes by:

1. describing two cohorts of women with diabetes in terms of their attitudes to diabetes, their knowledge of diabetes, their self management behaviours, and their health outcomes,
2. exploring the correlation between knowledge of diabetes, self-management and health outcomes, and
3. identifying factors associated with higher levels of diabetes knowledge

Method

The Australian Longitudinal Study on Women's Health (ALSWH) Data

Women in this study are from a nationally representative sample that includes 13716 women who were aged 45-50 years (1946-51 cohort) and 12432 women aged 70-75 years (1921-26 cohort) when the study began in 1996. The women were randomly selected from the national health insurance database (Medicare) that includes all permanent residents of Australia regardless of age or income, with deliberate oversampling of women living in rural and remote areas. The recruitment protocol and response rates have been described elsewhere (Lee et al. 2005). Comparison with the 1996 Australian Census indicated the respondents were broadly representative of women in the same age groups with some over-representation of married and more highly educated women (Brown et al. 1999). Survey 2, the first follow-up, was in 1998 for the 1946-51 cohort and in 1999 for the older cohort. This research was approved by the University of Newcastle Human Research Ethics Committee.

Diabetes Care Substudy

In September 2001, a 16-page survey was mailed to 366 women from the 1946-51 cohort and 1008 women from the 1921-26 cohort who said in Survey 1 or Survey 2 that they had been diagnosed with diabetes. A protocol of mail and telephone reminders to increase response rates was followed (Dillman 1978). The content of the survey was based on items adapted from existing diabetes questionnaires in the published literature and the questions were pilot tested and modified where necessary following focus group discussions at urban and rural diabetes education centres. The survey was designed to measure the type and duration of diabetes, level and frequency of diabetes care including home blood glucose monitoring, foot and eye care, measurement of HbAlc, lipids, microalbuminuria and retinal screening, and access to diabetes-related health services such as nutrition advice, podiatry services and diabetes education services. Items were also included to measure emotional adjustment in women with diabetes. Some women in the ALSWH who had reported having diabetes were not sent the questionnaire (n=188 from 1946-51 cohort and n=443 from 1921-26 cohort) if they were known to be deceased or lost to follow up, were already participating in another targeted substudy (to minimise respondent burden), or had requested not to be in substudies.

Measures

The following variables have been included in this analysis:

Diabetes

Participants were asked in Survey 1 in 1996 whether a doctor had ever told them that they had diabetes. At Survey 2 (in 1998 for women in the 1946-51 cohort and 1999 for women in the 1921-26 cohort), participants were asked whether they had been diagnosed with diabetes since 1996. Women who responded 'yes' in either Survey 1 or Survey 2 were considered to have been diagnosed with diabetes.

Comorbidity
Whether they had ever been told by a doctor that they had any of a list of fourteen medical conditions, including hypertension and heart disease.

Self-Rated Health
Women were asked to rate their health, in general, as excellent, very good, good, fair or poor.

Body Mass Index
Measured as self-reported weight (kg) / height (m²).

Number of Different Types of Medication Used
How many different types of medication used in the last four weeks which were prescribed by a doctor.

Physical Activity
Categorised as adequate (at least 5 bouts of moderate activity per week, or 3 bouts of vigorous activity, or any combination of the two) or inadequate based on questions about frequency and intensity of physical activity (Brown et al. 2000).

Education
Classified as 'no formal qualifications', 'high school', 'trade/diploma' and 'tertiary' qualifications.

Area of Residence
Coded as urban or non-urban based on postcode of residence.

Attitudes to Diabetes
Items from the ATT39 scale to measure women's attitude to having diabetes were included in the substudy questionnaire (Dunn et al. 1986; Welsh, Smith and Wlakey 1992). Women were asked how strongly they felt about each statement on a five-point scale ranging from 'completely disagree' to 'completely agree'. Responses of 'completely agree' and 'agree' were combined to reflect agreement with the statement.

Diabetes Knowledge, Self-Management Behaviours and Health Outcomes

Responses to the Diabetes Care Substudy were used to derive scores to reflect knowledge of diabetes, self-management and health outcomes. The *knowledge* score ranged from 0-4 and assessed whether the woman had heard of HbA1c tests, knew the normal range for blood glucose, understood good control of diabetes based on blood test results and knew whether her current weight was harmful to her health (BMI>27 was regarded as potentially harmful). The *behaviour* score ranged from 0-3 where poor behaviour was defined as not testing sugar levels at least 2-6 times weekly, having a BMI of 30 or more and not trying to lose weight, not exercising and not believing in the need to be more active (when there is no medical condition preventing exercise). The *outcome* score ranged from 0-8 and assessed glucose control over the previous month, number of hypoglycaemic episodes in the past year, days in hospital in the past year, BMI and number and severity of complications of diabetes (from a list of ten conditions which included poor circulation to the feet or legs, kidney disease, stroke, gangrene, foot or legs ulcers). The three scores were coded so that higher scores on each scale reflect better knowledge, behavior and outcomes.

Statistical Analysis

Basic descriptive statistics were used to describe the two age groups of women in terms of their demographic characteristics and their diabetes-related attitudes, knowledge, behaviours and health outcomes. The correlations between summary scores for knowledge, behaviour and outcomes were assessed using Pearson correlation coefficients. The association between the summary scores and a range of demographic, health, social and health care utilisation variables was examined using chi-squared tests and one-way ANOVA. To further investigate the correlates of better knowledge, a new dichotomous variable was defined: good knowledge (score ≥ 3) and poor knowledge (score < 3). Logistic regression analysis was performed to determine which variables were associated with better knowledge among both cohorts of women. The explanatory variables that were significant in bivariate analyses were included in the multivariate model. All statistical analyses were performed using SAS statistical software (SAS Institute Inc. 1999).

Results

The response to the Diabetes Care Substudy was 92% (336/366) for women in the 1946-51 cohort and 76% (769/1008) for women in the 1921-26 cohort. One third of the 1946-51 cohort women (n=113) and 15% of the 1921-26 cohort women (n=114) who responded stated that they had only experienced gestational diabetes or that they were "borderline". A profile of some characteristics of the remaining 878 respondents by age group is shown in Table 1. Most of the women had Type II diabetes, and 31% of the women from the 1946-51 cohort and 40% of women from the 1921-26 cohort had had diabetes for more than ten years.

Table 1. Characteristics of women with diabetes from the 1946-51 and 1921-26 cohorts

		1946-51 cohort (50-55 yrs) (n=223) %	1921-26 cohort (75-80 yrs) (n=655) %
Area of residence	Urban	33	38
	Large rural centre	9	12
	Small rural centre	17	18
	Other rural / remote area	41	33
		100	100
Education	No formal qualifications	25	37
	School only	50	49
	Trade/diploma	19	11
	Tertiary	6	2
		100	100
Type of diabetes	Type I	10	8
	Type II	90	92
		100	100

Table 1 (Continued)

Duration of diabetes	< 5 years	29	30
	5-10 years	40	30
	10-20 years	22	28
	>20 years	9	12
		100	100
Current treatment	No Treatment	8	8
	Diet/exercise (no meds)	21	22
	Tablets (no insulin)	50	53
	Insulin	21	18
		100	100
Self-assessment of control in the past year	Very well/Well controlled	46	64
	Average control	37	29
	Very poor/Poorly controlled	13	4
	Variable control	2	3
	Don't know	2	1
		100	100

In both age groups, most women expressed positive attitudes regarding the impact of diabetes on their lifestyle and their adjustment to having the condition (Table 2). However, 35% of the women from the 1946-51 cohort (and 26% of women from the 1921-26 cohort) believed that the proper control of diabetes involves a lot of sacrifice and inconvenience. Furthermore, around 35% of the women in both age groups did not like being told what to eat, when to eat, and how much. One-fifth of the women said they try not to let people know they have diabetes.

Table 2. Percentage of women who agree with positive and negative statements about having diabetes

Item	1946-51 cohort (50-55 yrs) (n=223)	1921-26 cohort (75-80 yrs) (n=655)
Positive statements	%	%
I believe I have adjusted well to having diabetes	79	86
Diabetes is not really a problem because it can be controlled	70	85
Having diabetes has encouraged me to improve my lifestyle	69	71
My diabetic diet does not really spoil my social life	68	62
Negative statements		
I try not to let people know about my diabetes	22	21
Most doctors really don't understand what it's like to have diabetes	27	19
The proper control of diabetes involves a lot of sacrifice and inconvenience	35	26
I do not like being told what to eat, when to eat, and how much	36	35

In general both groups of women had less than optimum levels of knowledge, and a large proportion did not engage in appropriate behaviours and preventive activities (Table 3). Although most of the older women understood the risk that being overweight had on their health, less than one-third were familiar with the HbA1c test and only half could correctly identify the normal range for blood glucose. The 1946-51 cohort women scored higher on the knowledge items but women in both age groups had similar responses to questions about how often they tested their blood glucose and the method used. Compared with women in the 1946-51 cohort, women from the 1921-26 cohort were more likely to have received preventive services such as having their feet and eyes examined and they were also more likely to be taking multiple medications. Women from the 1946-51 cohort were more likely to be overweight than the older women but had lower rates of complications such as poor circulation, retinopathy and hospitalisation. However approximately half the women with diabetes in the 1946-51 cohort reported being treated for hypertension and had been diagnosed with high cholesterol or triglycerides. Around two-thirds of women in each age-group had attended a diabetes education centre. There were few differences by age group in the type of practitioners who manage the care of these women, with general practitioners most likely to be providing diabetes care.

The knowledge summary scores for women in the 1921-26 cohort were positively correlated with behaviour and outcomes scores, indicating that older women with better knowledge of diabetes self-management had better self-management (r=0.246, p<0.0001) and also had more favourable outcomes (i.e. better diabetes control, fewer complications and hospitalisations) (r=0.238, p<0.0001). However there was no correlation between current diabetes care behaviours and health outcomes (p=0.549). Among the older women, higher knowledge scores were associated in bivariate analysis with having more education (p=0.007), receiving multidisciplinary diabetes care (p=0.0002), receiving nutritional advice from a dietitian (p=0.005), having HbA1c tests (p<0.0001) and eye tests (p<0.0001), and having visited a diabetes education centre (p<0.0001). Higher behaviour scores (better behaviour) were associated with having Type I diabetes (p=0.002), receiving care from a specialist (p<0.0001) and/or multidisciplinary care (p=0.0002), receiving nutrition advice (p=0.0003) and having visited a diabetes education centre (p=0.0004). In the multivariate logistic regression model, the significant predictors of better knowledge were having attended a diabetes education centre (odds ratio 2.04, 95% CI 1.33, 3.13) and having had a HbA1c test in the previous year (odds ratio 2.13, 95% CI 1.63, 2.78).

The knowledge scores for women from the 1946-51 cohort were positively correlated with behaviour scores, indicating that women with better knowledge of diabetes self-management had better self-management (r=0.273, p<0.0001). However neither knowledge nor behaviour scores were correlated with the summary health outcomes score among 1946-51 cohort women, possibly due to the lower prevalence of poor health outcomes and the time lag required for the development of complications of diabetes.

Among women from the 1946-51 cohort, higher knowledge scores were associated in bivariate analysis with having HbA1c (p<0.0001) and eye tests (p<0.0001), and having visited a diabetes education centre (p=0.002).

Table 3. Knowledge, behaviours and outcomes among women with diabetes from the 1946-51 and 1921-26 cohorts

	1946-51 cohort (50-55 yrs) (n=223)	1921-26 cohort (75-80 yrs) (n=655)
	%	%
Knowledge		
Heard of HbA1c (long term sugar) test	57	29
Knew normal range for blood glucose	72	49
Understood risk of overweight to health	71	76
Understood good control of diabetes	65	68
Behaviour		
Sugar levels tested at least 2-6 times weekly	63	59
Blood tested by meter at home	84	78
Taking more than seven medications	9	24
BMI $\geq$ 30	61	24
Preventive activities		
Feet examined in past year	58	72
Back of eyes examined in past year	53	62
Attended a diabetes education centre	66	66
Health Outcomes		
Blood tests mainly 4-10 mmol/L past month	61	68
More than one hypoglycaemic episode in past year	8	5
More than 7 days in hospital in last year	7	16
Currently being treated for hypertension	51	67
Ever had high cholesterol/triglycerides	48	50
Poor circulation to the feet/legs	18	43
Suffered from/treated for retinopathy	13	25
Had heart bypass surgery	2	9
Providers of diabetes care		
General practitioner	86	85
Diabetes specialist	31	26
Nurse/health worker	9	12
Multidisciplinary care	27	25

Higher behaviour scores were associated with having Type I diabetes (p=0.002), having HbA1c (p=0.004) and eye tests (p=0.003), having more frequent consultations with a GP (p=0.0007) and having attended a diabetes education centre (p=0.0045). In the multivariate logistic regression model, the significant predictors of better knowledge were having attended a diabetes education centre (odds ratio 2.45, 95% CI 1.14, 5.31) and having had a HbA1c test in the previous year (odds ratio 2.78, 95% CI 1.57, 4.91).

Discussion

Our study examined the knowledge of diabetes and the self-management of a random and representative sample of Australian women using a self-administered questionnaire. The results showed that at a community level there is a great need to improve knowledge and behaviours among the growing population of people with diabetes, particularly those with Type II diabetes. In this study, better knowledge was correlated with better behaviours (in both age groups) and with better health outcomes (among older women). In the logistic regression models, better knowledge was associated with having attended a diabetes education centre, providing strong support for the work of these centres.

The lower scores on knowledge and self-management among the older women in our study showed that women in this age group have a particular need for diabetes education. Although it has been estimated that 40% of people with diabetes are aged over 65 years, longitudinal trials of aspects of care have not routinely included these patients (Huang, Gorawara-Bhat and Chin 2004). It is also recognized that special factors must be considered for providing self-management education for older people with diabetes (American Association of Diabetes Educators 2003). It has been suggested that proactive management of patients with diabetes requires an interdisciplinary approach with the expertise and cooperation of several healthcare professionals. In this study, around 25% of women reported receiving such multi-disciplinary care.

In vulnerable populations, such as older people with chronic disease, there may be socioeconomic or geographic disparities in access to care (Young, Dobson and Byles 2000). However in this study, educational qualifications and geographical remoteness were not found to be associated with knowledge about diabetes nor with self-management, for each age cohort. Although the older women had lower knowledge about diabetes than the 1946-51 cohort women, they were more likely to have received preventive care such as having their feet and eyes examined. This finding is important as over half the diabetes-related lower-extremity amputations may be prevented with regular foot examinations and patient education (Valente, Caughy and Fischbach 2004).

Our study has a number of limitations. Firstly data are unavailable to determine whether these findings are consistent for men in Australia, as the longitudinal study was commissioned to explore the factors contributing to the health of women. Second, women with poor education are slightly under-represented in the study (Brown et al. 1999) and so the sample may be biased towards the higher end of the range of health literacy. Third, the survey may be measuring how well women understand the information and recommendations provided by their health care providers, rather than measuring the education and care that was offered. However the advantage of this study is that it is based on a large random sample of women rather than the convenience samples that are often used when studying chronic illness.

Conclusion

Complications of diabetes are taking an increasing toll on public health resources, and the prevention and treatment of complications are primary goals of public health initiatives. To reach these goals, each person requires consistent care, preferably a team of professionals working together. This study found that attending diabetes education centres and having higher levels of knowledge of diabetes management was associated with better self-management behaviours and potentially better health outcomes for women with diabetes. The findings on the perceived impact of diabetes and its treatment on the lifestyle of the women may inform strategies for intervention among those women with poor management of their diabetes. Although many women had access to preventive care and screening services for their diabetes, further strategies are needed to improve knowledge about diabetes, self-care behaviour and health outcomes, particularly for older women.

Acknowledgments

The Australian Longitudinal Study on Women's Health, which is conducted by researchers at the Universities of Newcastle and Queensland, is funded by the Australian Government Department of Health and Ageing. This research was also supported by a Diabetes Australia Research Trust grant. We thank Amanda Patterson for her contribution to planning the project, Jane Watson for managing the Diabetes Care Substudy and Virginia Wheway for assisting with statistical analysis. Finally we thank all participants for their valuable contribution to this project.

References

American Association of Diabetes Educators. Special considerations for the education and management of older adults with diabetes. *The Diabetes Educator*. 2003; 29: 93-95.

Beckles, G.L.A., Engelau, M.M., Vencat Narayan, K.M., Herman, W.H., Aubert, R.E., Williamson, D.F. Population-based assessment of the level of care among adults with diabetes in the US. *Diabetes Care*. 1998; 21: 1432-1438.

Brown, W.J., Bryson, L., Byles, J.E., Dobson, A.J., Lee, C., Mishra, G., Schofield, M. Women's Health Australia: Recruitment for a national longitudinal cohort study. *Women & Health*. 1998; 28: 23-40.

Brown, W.J., Dobson, A.J., Bryson, L., Byles, J.E. Women's Health Australia: on the progress of the main study cohorts. *Journal of Women's Health & Gender-based Medicine*. 1999; 8: 681-688.

Brown, W.J., Mishra, G., Lee, C., Bauman, A. Leisure time physical activity in Australian women: relationship with well being and symptoms. *Res Q Exercise Sport*. 2000; 71: 206-216.

Corser, W. Facilitating patients' diabetes self-management: A primary care intervention framework. *J Nursing Care Quality*, 2009; 24(2):172-178.

Deakin TA, McShane CE, Cade JE, Williams R. Group based training for self-management strategies in people with type 2 diabetes mellitus. *Cochrane Database of Systematic Reviews* 2005, Issue 2. Art. No.: CD003417. DOI: 10.1002/14651858.CD003417.pub2.

Dillman, D.A. Mail and telephone surveys: The total design method. New York: Wiley, 1978.

Dunn, S.M., Smartt, H.H., Beeney, L.J., Turtle, J.R. Measurement of emotional adjustment in diabetic patients: validity and reliability of ATT39. *Diabetes Care*. 1986; 9: 480-489.

Diabetes Australia and the Royal Australian College of General Practitioners: Diabetes management in general practice. Eleventh edition. Canberra, Diabetes Australia, 2005.
http://www.racgp.org.au/downloads/pdf/20051114diabetesbooklet.pdf

Fleming, B.B., Greenfield, S., Engelgau, M.M., et al. The Diabetes Quality Improvement Project. *Diabetes Care*, 2001; 24:1815–1820.

Funnell, M.M., and Anderson, R.M. Empowerment and self-management of diabetes. *Clinical Diabetes*, 2004; 22:123–128.

Giugliano, D,. Standl, E,. Vilsboll, T,. Betteridge, J,. Bonadonna, R,. Campbell, I.W., Schernthaner, G.H., Staels, B., Trichopoulou, A., Farinaro, E. Is the current therapeutic armamentarium in diabetes enough to control the epidemic and its consequences? What are the current shortcomings? *Acta Diabetologica*. 46(3):173-81, 2009.

Heisler, M., Smith, D.M., Hayward, R.A., Krein, S.L., Kerr, E.A. How well do patients' assessments of their diabetes self-management correlate with actual glycemic control and receipt of recommended diabetes services? *Diabetes Care*. 2003; 26: 738-743.

Huang, E.S, Gorawara-Bhat, R. and Chin, M.H. Practical challenges of individualizing diabetes care in older patients. *The Diabetes Educator*. 2004; 30: 558-570.

Jorgensen, W.A., Polivka, B.J., Lennie, T.A. Perceived adherence to prescribed or recommended standards of care among adults with diabetes. *The Diabetes Educator*. 2002; 28: 989-998.

Keers, J.C., Bouma, J., Links, T.P., et al. One-year follow-up effects of diabetes rehabilitation for patients with prolonged self-management difficulties. *Patient Educ Couns*. 2006;60(1):16–23.

Lee, C., Dobson, A.J., Brown, W.J., Bryson, L., Byles, J., Warner-Smith, P., Young, A.F. Cohort Profile: The Australian Longitudinal Study on Women's Health. *International Journal of Epidemiology*. 2005; 34: 987-991.

Nagelkerk, J., Reick, K. and Meengs, L. Perceived barriers and effective strategies to diabetes self-management. *J Adv Nurs*. 2006;54(2):151–158.

Nasmith, L., Cote, B., Cox, J., et al. The challenge of promoting integration: conceptualization, implementation, and assessment of a pilot care delivery model for patients with type 2 diabetes. *Fam Med.* 004;36(1):40–45.

Oosthuizen, H., Riedijik, R., Nonner, J., et al. An educational intervention to improve the quality of care of diabetic patients. *South African Medical Journal.* 2002; 92: 459–464.

Peyrot, M., Rubin, R.R., Lauritzen, T., et al. Patient and provider perceptions of care for diabetes: results of the cross-national DAWN study. *Diabetologia.* 2006;49(2):279–288.

Saaddine, J.B., Engelgau,M.M., Beckles, G.L., et al. A diabetes report card for the United States: quality of care in the 1990s. *Ann Intern Med.* 2002; 136:565-574.

Saaddine, J.B., Cadwell, B., Gregg, E.W., Engelgau, M.M., Vinicor, F., Imperatore, G. and Narayan, K.M. Improvements in diabetes processes of care and intermediate outcomes: United States, 1988-2002. *Ann Intern Med.* 2006; 144(7): 465-74.

Salas, M., Hughes, D., Zuluaga, A., Vardeva, K. and Lebmeier, M. Costs of medication nonadherence in patients with diabetes mellitus: a systematic review and critical analysis of the literature. *Value in Health.* 2009; 12(6):915-22.

SAS Institute Inc. SAS/STAT User's guide, Version 8. Cary, NC, SAS Institute Inc., 1999.

Seley, J.J. and Weinger, K. Executive summary: the state of the science on nursing best practices for diabetes self-management. *Am J Nurs.* 2007;107(6):73–78.

Setter, S.M., Corbett, C.F., Campbell, R.K., Cook, D. and Gates, B.J. A survey of the perceptions, knowledge, and use of A1C values by home care patients and nurses. *The Diabetes Educator.* 2003; 29: 144-152.

Tomky, D.M. Developing a computerized diabetes self-management education module for documenting outcomes. *The Diabetes Educator.* 1999; 25: 197-209.

Valente, L.A., Caughy, M. and Fischbach, L. A validation study of a self-administered questionnaire to identify increased risk for foot ulceration or amputation among people with diabetes. *The Diabetes Educator.* 2004; 30: 932-944.

Welsh, G., Smith, B.W. and Walkey, F.H. Styles of psychological adjustment in diabetes: a focus on key psychometric issues and the ATT39. *Journal of Clinical Psychology.* 1992; 48: 648-658.

Young, A.F., Lowe, J.M., Byles, J.E., Patterson, A.J. Trends in health service use for women in Australia with diabetes. *Australian and New Zealand Journal of Public Health*. 2005; 29: 422-428.

Young, A.F., Dobson, A.J. and Byles, J.E. Access and equity in the provision of general practitioner services in Australia. *Australian and New Zealand Journal of Public Health*. 2000; 24: 474-480.

In: Diabetes in Women   ISBN: 978-1-61668-692-5
Editor: Eliza I. Swahn, pp. 67-82   © 2010 Nova Science Publishers, Inc.

Chapter IV

Early Mortality in Diabetic Women with Non-ST Elevation Myocardial Infarction

*Andreja Sinkovic**

University Medical Centre Maribor, Department of medical intensive care,
SI-2000 Maribor, Slovenia

Abstract

Background. In contrast to ST elevation myocardial infarcts in non-ST-elevation myocardial infarction (NSTEMI) prognosis in women and men are equal and in unstable angina even in favour of women compared to men. Diabetes is common amongst patients admitted with NSTEMI, in particular in women as demonstrated by several clinical trials. Diabetic in comparison with non diabetic patients with NSTEMI in general have more clinical complications, increased mortality, longer in-hospital stay

* Correspondence:
Andreja Sinkovic
University Medical Centre Maribor
Department of medical intensive care
Ljubljanska 5
SI-2000 Maribor, Slovenia
E-mail: Andreja.sinkovic@guest.arnes.si

and increased management costs. However, the prognosis in diabetic women in comparison to their diabetic counterparts, diabetic and nondiabetic men with NSTEMI is less well known. Our aim was to evaluate and compare 30-day mortality between diabetic and nondiabetic women, diabetic women and diabetic and nondiabetic men with NSTEMI.

Patients and Methods

We retrospectively analysed all the records of patients discharged with the diagnosis NSTEMI during one year period. 415 patients, 181 women (mean age 71,2 ± 11,9 years), 234 men (mean age 64.8 ± 10.8 years) fullfilled the inclusion criteria, being rest chest pain, lasting up to 48 hours before addmission, ECG changes without ST-elevation, but with ST-depression and/or negative T wave and increase in Troponin T, estimated by immunochemical method (normal levels up to 0.1μg/l), suggesting the size of ischemic necrosis. The patients were treated by antiplatelet, anticoagulant therapy and percutaneous coronary intervention. During 30-day follow-up demographic data, in particular diabetes, and 30-day mortality were registered.

Results

Diabetes was observed in 24.3% of patients with NSTEMI. Between the genders there was a nonsignificant difference in the incidence of diabetes, being 22.8% in women and 25.7% in men. Mean admission troponin T level was 0.38 ± 0.7μg/l and peak Troponin T 0.82 ± 1.3μg/l. There were nonsignificant differences in mean peak Troponin T levels between diabetic and nondiabetic patients (0.81 ± 1.6μg/l vs 0.8 ± 1.2μg/l), diabetic and nondiabetic women (1.2 ± 2.0μg/l vs 0.81 ± 1.2μg/l), diabetic women and nondiabetic men (1.2 ± 2.0μg/l vs 0.82 ± 1.3μg/l) and diabetic women and men (1.2 ± 2.0μg/l vs 0.56 ± 0.9μg/l). 30-day mortality of patients with NSTEMI was 4.3%. Any significant differences were observed in overall 30-day mortality between men and women (3.0% vs 9.3%), neither between diabetics and nondiabetics with NSTEMI (5.9% vs 3.8%), between diabetic and nondiabetic women (6.9% vs 5.5%), nondiabetic men and nondiabetic women (2.4% vs 5.5%) and between diabetic men and women (5.2% vs 6.9%).

Conclusion

30-day mortality in diabetic women with NSTEMI is similar to nondiabetic patients with NSTEMI, either men or women.

Background

Diabetes mellitus (DM) is one of the major risk factors for coronary artery disease and at the same time many patients with known or symptomatic coronary artery disease suffer from DM and its complications (1-5). DM is defined as chronic hyperglicaemia with disturbed carbohydrate, fat and protein metabolism. It is the consequence of either a defect in insulin secretion, or insulin action, or both. Therefore in DM type 1 there is a complete lack of endogenous pancreatic insulin production, but in DM type 2 resistence to insulin action mostly predominates (5, 6). In long-term, DM predisposes to organ damages, in particular cardio-vascular, cerebrovascular and peripheral artery disease (5-7).

The diagnosis of DM is based on fasting and postprandial plasma glucose levels. According to WHO fasting plasma glucose level over 7 mmol/l and two-hour post-load plasma glucose over 11.1 mmol/L are the criteria for DM (5, 6, 8).

In diabetic patients the risk for coronary artery disease is 2-3-times increased and cardiovascular diseases are most important cause of death in both types of DM (5, 9-11).

According to the results of GRACE registry from 2003 the overall incidence of DM in patients with acute coronary syndromes was approximately 20%, but it was 21% in patients with ST-elevation myocardial infarction and 25% with NSTEMI (1). Epidemiology data on acute coronary syndromes some years later revealed an increase in the incidence of DM to 28% in ST-elevation MI patients, but in NSTEMI patients the incidence of DM remained the same – 21% (2).

Several clinical studies demonstrated that DM is more common in women than in men with NSTEMI (12). Regarding some some clinical studies diabetic patients with NTEMI in comparison to non-diabetic counterparts have more clinical complications in general, in particular increased mortality, longer in-hospital stay and increased management costs (3-5,10,). Regarding NSTEMI prognosis such as in-hospital mortality is equal in men and women and in unstable angina prognosis is even in favour of women compared to men (13-15). However, the prognosis in diabetic women in comparison to their diabetic counterparts, diabetic and nondiabetic men with NSTEMI is less well known . Our aim was to evaluate and compare 30-day mortality between diabetic and nondiabetic women, diabetic women and diabetic and nondiabetic men with NSTEMI.

Patients and Methods

We retrospectively analysed the records of all the patients, admitted and discharged between January 1st 2006 and December 31st 2006 at the University clinical centre Maribor due to acute myocardial infarction. All the data were obtained by the hospital computer programme Medis. Finally, we included only 415 patients (227 men, 188 women, mean age 67.69 ± 11.77 years), meeting the criteria for NSTEMI. The inclusion criteria were oppressive chest pain at rest, lasting up to 48 hours before admission and ECG changes, consisting of ST-segment depression ≥ 0,1 mV and/or ST-segment depression with slight ST-segment elevation and/or negative T wave ≥ 0,1 mV and/or pathologic Q wave suspective of previous myocardial infarction and/or non-specific changes on ECG with elevated troponin T levels (7,16,17).

In patients standard ECG was recorded on admission, every 24 hours of hospital stay and at recurrent chest pain. Serum Troponin T (TnT) levels were estimated by immunochemical method (Boehringer, Mannheim – Germany, normal levels up to 0.1 µg/L) on admission, 8 and 24 hours later and at the discretion of the attending physician, particularly in case of recurrent chest pain (7,16,17). On admission plasma the lipid profile was estimated - total cholesterol, triglycerides, HDL-cholesterol and LDL-cholesterol levels by standard enzymatic methods (Olympus – Japan).

Acute ischemic necrosis – NSTEMI was confirmed by an increase in TnT level > 0.1 µg/L either on admission and/or 8-12 hours later (17).

Patients received daily oral acetylsalycylic acid (ASA) (100-300 mg tablet), i.v. infusion of standard heparin (SH) or s.c. injection of the recommended dose of low molecular weight heparin (LMWH) for few days, that was prolonged at the discretion of the attending physician (7). If necessary, the patients were treated by nitroglycerin, clopidogrel, beta-blockers, ACE inhibitors, statins, diuretics, calcium antagonists, dobutamin, norepinephrin, dopamine, levosimendan, intraaortic-baloon counterpulsation, etc. (7,16,18, 20,21).

In case of recurrent chest pain and/or hemodynamic instability and/or rhythmic instability within the first 48 hours, the patients were treated with glycoprotein receptor antagonists IIb/IIIa (tirofiban, integrillin, abciximab), followed by early percutaneous coronary angiography and intervention (PCI) or surgical revascularization (7,20). PCI was associated with clopidogrel therapy - loading dose 300 mg, followed by 75 mg daily (7, 20, 21). When the patients were asymptomatic during the first 48 hours, coronary angiography with subsequent PCI or surgical revascularization was performed later within the next few days or weeks, in particular if ischemia was detected by exercise testing (7,20).

In all the patients we detected demographic, clinical and laboratory data, including age, previous arterial hypertension, diabetes, prior myocardial infarction and/or stroke, smoking, troponin T levels, serum creatinine on admission and during in-hospital stay as well as admission lipid profile, in-hospital heart failure and 30-day mortality. In-hospital heart failure was defined according to Killip-Kimball classification. Patients with heart failure belonged to Killip classes II, III and IV (18,19).

The patients were grouped according to gender and the diagnosis of previous DM into several groups. The diagnosis of previous DM was based on WHO criteria, considering fasting and two-hour post-load plasma glucose levels, where fasting plasma glucose level exceeded 7 mmol/l and on two-hour post-load plasma glucose 11.1 mmol/L (8). We compared diabetic and nondiabetic patients with NSTEMI, diabetic men and women, nondiabetic men and women and finally nondiabetic and diabetic women with NSTEMi regarding the demographic, clinical and laboratory dat, but in particular 30-day mortality.

Statistical Analysis

The retrospectively collected data were analyzed using SPSS for Windows with basic statistical methods. The values were expressed as means ± standard deviations, or percentages. The differences between the groups were tested using chi-square test and two-sided Student's t-test. Values $p < 0.05$ were considered statistically significant (22).

Results

Demographic, clinical and laboratory data of our NSTEMI patients are displayed in Table 1. 54.7% of patients were men and 45.3% were women. DM was present in 24.3% of our NSTEMI patients. Out of the diabetic patients 57.4% were men and 42.6% were women. Between the genders there was a nonsignificant difference in the incidence of DM.

Table 1. Demographic, clinical and laboratory data of all the patients with non-ST-elevation myocardial infarction

Demographic, clinical and laboratory data	Patients (n = 415)
Men / women (% men)	227 / 188 (54.7)
Age ± SD (years)	67.7 ± 11.8
Prior MI (%)	29.4
Prior stroke (%)	7.5
Arterial hypertension (%)	83.1
Smoking (%)	15.2
Troponin T ± SD (µg/l)	0.4 ± 0.7
Total serum-cholesterol ± SD (mmo/l)	4.9 ± 1.3
HDL-cholesterol ± SD (mmo/l)	1.1 ± 0.3
LDL-cholesterol ± SD (mmo/l)	2.9 ± 1.0
Triglicerides ± SD (mmo/l)	1.97 ± 1.5
Diabetes (%)	24.3
Admission creatinine ± SD (µmol/l)	108.0 ± 98.4
Admisssion heart failure (%)	10.4
Peak troponin T ± SD (µg/l)	0.82 ± 1.3
Peak serum creatinine ± SD (µmol/l)	124.8 ± 125.6
In-hospital heart failure (%)	10.1
30-day mortality (%)	4.3

Comparisons of demographic, clinical and laboratory data between diabetic and nondiabetic NSTEMI patients are displayed in Table 2, between diabetic men and women in Table 3, between nondiabetic men and women in Table 4 and between diabetic and nondiabetic women in Table 5.

Table 2. Comparison of demographic, clinical and laboratory data between the diabetic and nondiabetic patients with non-ST-elevation myocardial infarction

Demographic, clinical, laboratory data	Diabetics (n = 101)	Nondiabetics (n = 314)	p
Men / women (% men)	58 /43 (57.4)	169 / 145 (53.8)	0.605
Age ± SD (years)	69.0 ± 10.5	67.3 ± 12.1	0.206
Prior MI (%)	36.6	27.1	0.092
Prior stroke (%)	11.9	6.1	0.090
Arterial hypertension (%)	96.0	79.0	< 0.001
Smoking (%)	10.9	16.6	0.223
Troponin T ± SD (µg/l)	0.3 ± 0.8	0.4 ± 0.6	0.285
Total serum-cholesterol ± SD (mmo/l)	4.6 ± 1.2	4.98 ± 1.4	0.014
HDL-cholesterol ± SD (mmo/l)	1.0 ± 0.22	1.2 ± 0.3	< 0.001
LDL-cholesterol ± SD (mmo/l)	2.6 ± 1.0	2.95 ± 1.0	0.002
Triglicerides ± SD (mmo/l)	2.2 ± 1.22	1.9 ± 1.6	0.084
Admission creatinine ± SD (µmol/l)	109.4 ± 63.0	107.6 ± 107.5	0.873
Admisssion heart failure (%)	11.9	9.9	0.699
Peak troponin T ± SD (µg/l)	0.81 ± 1.6	0.8 ± 1.2	0.893
Peak serum creatinine ± SD (µmol/l)	123.4 ± 74.6	125.3 ± 138.2	0.895
In-hospital heart failure (%)	12.9	9.2	0.380
30-day mortality (%)	5.9	3.8	0.537

Legend: SD, standard deviation; MI, myocardial infarction; HDL, high-density lipoprotein; LDL, low-density lipoprotein

Table 3. Comparison of demographic, clinical and laboratory data between diabetic men and women with non ST-elevation myocardial infarction

Demographic, clinical, laboratory data	Men (n = 58)	Women (n = 43)	p
Age ± SD (years)	65.7 ± 10.99	73.5 ± 8.0	< 0.001
Prior MI (%)	43.1	27.9	0.098
Prior stroke (%)	12.6	11.6	1.000
Arterial hypertension (%)	96.6	95.3	0.576
Smoking (%)	8.9	4.7	0.108
Troponin T ± SD (µg/l)	0.23 ± 0.6	0.5 ± 0.93	0.144
Total serum-cholesterol ± SD (mmo/l)	4.7 ± 1.3	4.5 ± 1.2	0.489
HDL-cholesterol ± SD (mmo/l)	1.0 ± 0.23	1.0 ± 0.22	0.463
LDL-cholesterol ± SD (mmo/l)	2.7 ± 0.99	2.5 ± 1.0	0.585
Triglicerides ± SD (mmo/l)	2.2 ± 1.3	2.0 ± 1.0	0.547
Admission creatinine ± SD (µmol/l)	109.7 ± 64.4	108.98 ± 62.0	0.957
Admisssion heart failure (%)	13.8	9.3	0.551
Peak troponin T ± SD (µg/l)	0.56 ± 0.9	1.2 ± 2.0	0.060
Peak serum creatinine ± SD (µmol/l)	123.6 ± 79.4	123.0 ± 68.6	0.967
In-hospital heart failure (%)	12.0	13.9	0.774
30-day mortality (%)	5.2	6.9	0.698

Legend: SD, standard deviation; MI, myocardial infarction; HDL, high-density lipoprotein; LDL, low-density lipoprotein

Table 4. Comparison of demographic, clinical and laboratory data between nondiabetic men and women with non-ST-elevation myocardial infarction

Demographic, clinical, laboratory data	Men (n = 169)	Women (n = 145)	p
Age ± SD (years)	64.4 ± 10.8	70.5 ± 12.8	< 0.001
Prior MI (%)	27.2	26.9	1.000
Prior stroke (%)	4.1	8.3	0.155
Arterial hypertension (%)	76.9	81.4	0.562
Smoking (%)	24.9	6.9	< 0.001
Troponin T ± SD (µg/l)	0.4 ± 0.6	0.4 ± 0.6	0.940
Total serum-cholesterol ± SD (mmo/l)	4.8 ± 1.3	5.2 ± 1.4	0.020
HDL-cholesterol ± SD (mmo/l)	1.0 ± 0.3	1.2 ± 0.3	< 0.001
LDL-cholesterol ± SD (mmo/l)	2.8 ± 1.0	3.1 ± 1.0	0.039
Triglicerides ± SD (mmo/l)	1.96 ± 1.8	1.8 ± 1.2	0.520
Admission creatinine ± SD (µmol/l)	112.9 ± 121.2	101.5 ± 89.1	0.352
Admisssion heart failure (%)	8.3	11.7	0.347
Peak troponin T ± SD (µg/l)	0.82 ± 1.3	0.81 ± 1.2	0.927
Peak serum creatinine ± SD (µmol/l)	130.5 ± 149.3	119.2 ± 124.4	0.472
In-hospital heart failure (%)	8.3	10.3	0.562
30-day mortality (%)	2.4	5.5	0.237

Legend: SD, standard deviation; MI, myocardial infarction; HDL, high-density lipoprotein; LDL, low-density lipoprotein

There were nonsignificant differences in mean peak Troponin T levels between diabetic and nondiabetic patients (0.81 ± 1.6µg/l vs 0.8 ± 1.2µg/l), diabetic and nondiabetic women (1.2 ± 2.0µg/l vs 0.81 ± 1.2µg/l), diabetic women and nondiabetic men (1.2 ± 2.0µg/l vs 0.82 ± 1.3µg/l) and diabetic women and men (1.2 ± 2.0µg/l vs 0.56 ± 0.9µg/l).

Table 5. Comparison of demographic, clinical and laboratory data between nondiabetic and diabetic women with non-ST-elevation myocardial infarction

Demographic, clinical, laboratory data	Nondiabetic women (n = 145)	Diabetic women (n = 43)	p
Age ± SD (years)	70.5 ± 12.8	73.5 ± 8.0	0.147
Prior MI (%)	26.9	27.9	0.948
Prior stroke (%)	8.3	11.6	0.722
Arterial hypertension (%)	81.4	95.3	0.048
Smoking (%)	6.9	4.7	0.877
Troponin T ± SD (µg/l)	0.4 ± 0.6	0.5 ± 0.93	0.404
Total serum-cholesterol ± SD (mmo/l)	5.2 ± 1.4	4.5 ± 1.2	0.003
HDL-cholesterol ± SD (mmo/l)	1.2 ± 0.3	1.0 ± 0.22	< 0.001
LDL-cholesterol ± SD (mmo/l)	3.1 ± 1.0	2.5 ± 1.0	< 0.001
Triglicerides ± SD (mmo/l)	1.8 ± 1.2	2.0 ± 1.0	0.321
Admission creatinine ± SD (µmol/l)	101.5 ± 89.1	108.98 ± 62.0	0.607
Admisssion heart failure (%)	11.7	9.3	0.877
Peak troponin T ± SD (µg/l)	0.81 ± 1.2	1.2 ± 2.0	0.115
Peak serum creatinine ± SD (µmol/l)	119.2 ± 124.4	123.0 ± 68.6	0.848
In-hospital heart failure (%)	10.3	13.9	0.701
30-day mortality (%)	5.5	6.9	0.980

Legend: SD, standard deviation; MI, myocardial infarction; HDL, high-density lipoprotein; LDL, low-density lipoprotein

30-day mortality of patients with NSTEMI was 4.3%. Any significant differences were observed in overall 30-day mortality between men and women (3.0% vs 9.3%), neither between diabetics and nondiabetics with NSTEMI (5.9% vs 3.8%), between diabetic and nondiabetic women (6.9% vs 5.5%), nondiabetic men and nondiabetic women (2.4% vs 5.5%) nor between diabetic men and women (5.2% vs 6.9%).

Discussion

Our results suggest that 30-day mortality in diabetic women with NSTEMI is similar to early mortality in nondiabetic patients, either men or women.

The incidence of DM in our patients with NSTEMI was 24.3%, what is similar to the results of GRACE registry in 1999/2000, being 25% (1). However, the results of GRACE registry in 2005 demonstrated an increase in DM to 28% in NSTEMI patients (2).

In majority of registries NSTEMI predominates in males (1, 2, 23-25). In GRACE registry 63 – 65% of patients were males (2). However, in our NSTEMI population the difference in genders was nonsignificant as men accounted for 54.7% and women for 45.3% of the admitted population. The same was true for our diabetic subpopulation - gender difference remained nonsignificant as men accounted for 57.4% and women for 42.6% of cases. However, we observed significant age differences as our diabetic and nondiabetic women with NSTEMI were significantly older than their male counterparts. In spite of older age, 30-day mortality in women, either with or without DM was similar as in men. In addition, mortality was similar between diabetic and nondiabetic women, in whome there was a nonsignificant age difference.

In spite of older age in diabetic women their admission and peak troponin T levels, the lipid profile, the incidence of other prior chronic diseases as well as admission and in-hospital heart failure and 30-day mortality were similar as in diabetic men. On the other hand between nondiabetic men and women there was a significant difference in the mean serum lipid levels, being significantly higher in women than in men. However, in nondiabetic women we observed significantly increased mean HDL-cholesterol in comparison to men, which is protective in coronary artery disease.

Our results regarding the early outcome in diabetic women with NSTEMI are encouraging. Our data confirm the results of several prospective studies of invasive therapy in acute coronary syndrome patients, demonstrating that coronary artery disease is less severe in women than in men as there are significantly less severe stenotic coronary lesions and less extensive atherosclerosis changes of the coronary arteries in women than in men, in particular in NSTEMI (15, 26-28). However, more clinical studies, that would include women with NSTEMI, should be performed to give better understanding and more objective results. (29)

Comparing 30-day mortality among different groups according to gender and DM it seems that DM in women with NSTEMI did not exert any significant impact on 30-day mortality.

Irrespective of gender in our NSTEMI patients DM was not associated with either significantly increased early mortality nor heart failure. These finding are different to other clinical studies, demonstating that in-hospital complications such as heart failure and in-hospital mortality were more frequent in diabetic patients, in particular with other concommitant chronic conditions such as arterial hypertension (3,4,9). In our diabetic patients arterial hypertension was an imortant concommitant chronic disease, present in even more than 90% of our diabetics. However, arterial hypertension was very frequent in all subgroups of patients and in particular in diabetic women. According to studies the coexistence of diabetes and hypertension represents an important risk factor for adverse outcome of NSTEMI patients in general as it usually doubles the risk of adverse outcome in these patients (10). In spite of high incidence of arterial hypertension in our diabetic women their 30-day mortality was nonsignificantly increased in comparison to nondiabetic men and women, as well as diabetic men.

We observe significantly increased mean levels of total serum cholesterol, LDL- and HDL-cholesterol in nondiabetic women in comparison to diabetic ones. DM usually induces the increase in LDL-cholesterol and triglicerides and decrease in HDL-cholesterol (5). We speculate that decreased levels in our diabetic women could be the consequence of prior antidiabetic therapy, either by insulin or oral antidiabetic drugs, which improve the lipid profile.

Mean admission and peak troponin levels in diabetic women were similar to troponin levels in all the groups of NSTEMI patients, reflecting similar magnitude of ischemic necrosis, resulting in similar prognosis such as similar incidence of in-hospital heart failure and 30-day mortality (24).

According to studies, the initial uncomplicated 30-day outcome in NSTEMI patients can be frequently followed by long-term increased mortality due to recurrent ischemia with reinfarction and due to heart failure (10). To avoid the risk of underestimating the long-term adverse outcome in spite of early uneventful course in NSTEMI accurate early assessment of left ventricular function such as ejection fraction and anatomy such as left ventricular dimensions should be performed and treatment by ACE inhibitors should be initiated to prevent remodelling in every patient after NSTEMI, particularly with DM – equally in men and women (7). HOPE (The Heart Outcome Prevention Evaluation), EUROPA (EURopean trial On reduction of cardiac events with Perindopril in stable coronary Artery) and other studies have clearly demonstrated the beneficial effect of ACE inhibition in all the patients with established arterial atherosclerosis irrespective of overt symptomatic heart failure or decreased ejection fraction (30-32).

In addition, early coronary angiography with subsequent coronary intervention or by pass grafting should be performed to solve any residual coronary ischemia and therefore to prevent reinfarction, subsequent heart failure and mortality in particularly in diabetic patients, women included equally (20).

Our conclusions are that in contemporary western civilisation there are any significant gender-related differences in hospital admissions for NSTEMI, resulting in similar outcome even in diabetic women with NSTEMI.

References

[1]   Fox KAA, Goodman SG, Anderson FA Jr, Granger CB, Moscucci M, Flather MD, Spence F, Budaj A, Dabbous O, Gore JM, on behalf of the GRACE Investigators. From Giudelines to clinical practice: The impact of hospital and geographic characteristics on temporal trends in the management of acute coronary syndroms. The Global Registry of Acute Coronary Events (GRACE). *Eur Heart J.* 2003; 24: 1414-24.

[2]   Fox KAA, Steg PG, Eagle KA, Goodman SG, Anderson FA, Granger CB in sod for the GARCE investigators. Decline in rates of death and heart failure in acute coronary syndromes, 1999-2006. *JAMA,* 2007; 297: 1892-900.

[3]   Bakhai A, Collinson J, Flather MD, de Arenaza DP, Shibata MC, Wang D, Adgey JA; KAA Fox for the PRAIS-UK Investigators. Diabetic patients with acute coronary syndromes in the UK: high risk and under treated. Results from the prospective registry of acute ischaemic syndromes in the UK (PRAIS-UK). *Int J Cardiol.* 2005; 100: 79-84.

[4]   Novo G, Scordato F, Cerruto G, Vitale G, Ciaramitaro G, Coppola G, Farinella M, Rotolo A, Indovina G, Assennato P, Novo S. In-hospital stay of patient with acute coronary syndrome with or without diabetes mellitus. *Minerva Cardioangiol* 2009; 57: 159-64.

[5]   Rydén L, Standl E, Bartnik M, Van den Berghe G, Betteridge J, de Boer M-J, Cosentino F, Jönsson B, Laakso M, Malmberg K, Priori S, Östergren J, Tuomilehto J and Thrainsdottir I. Guidelines on diabetes, pre-diabetes, and cardiovascular diseases: executive summary.

[6]   The Task Force on Diabetes and Cardiovascular Diseases of the European Society of Cardiology (ESC) and of the European Association for the Study of Diabetes (EASD). *Eur Heart J.* 2007; 28: 88-136.

[7]   Unwin N, Shaw J, Zimmet P, Alberti KG. Impaired glucose tolerance and impaired fasting glycaemia: the current status on definition and intervention. *Diabet Med* 2002; 19: 708-23.

[8]   Bassand JP, Hamm CW, Ardissino D, Boersma E, Budaj A, Fernandez-Aviles F, Fox KAA, Hasdai D, Ohman EM, Wallentin L, Wijns W. Non-ST-segment Elevation Acute Coronary Syndromes (Guidelines for the Diagnosis and Treatment of. *Eur Heart J.* 2008; 28: 1598-660.

[9]   WHO Consultation. Definition, diagnosis and classification of diabetes mellitus and its. Complications. Part 1: diagnosis and classification of diabetes mellitus. Geneva: World Health Organization; 1999. report no. 99.2.

[10] Farkouh ME, Aneja A, Reeder GS, Smars PA, Lennon RJ, Wiste HJ, Traverse K, Razzouk L, Basu A, Holmes DR Jr, Mathew V. Usefulness of diabetes mellitus to predict long-term outcomes in patients with unstable angina pectoris. *Am J Cardiol.* 2009; 104: 492-7.

[11] Colivicchi F, Mettimano M, Genovesi-Ebert A, Schinzari F, Iantorno M, Melina G, Santini M, Cardillo C, Melina D. Differences between diabetic and non-diabetic hypertensive patients with first acute non-ST elevation myocardial infarction and predictors of in-hospital complications. *J Cardiovasc Med.* 2008; 9: 267-7.

[12] Donahoe SM, Stewart GC, McCabe CH, Mohanavelu S, Murphy SA, Cannon CP, Antman EM. Diabetes and mortality following acute coronary syndromes. *JAMA.* 2007; 298: 765-75.1

[13] Heer T, Gitt AK, Juenger C, Schiele R, Wienbergen H, Towae F, Gottwitz M, Zahn R, Zeymer U, Senges J; ACOS Investigators. Gender differences in acute non-ST-segment elevation myocardial infarction. *Am J Cardiol.* 2006; 98: 160-6.

[14] Roger VL, Farkouh ME, Weston SA, et al. Sex differences in evaluation and outcome of unstable angina. *JAMA,* 2000; 283: 646-52.

[15] Sinkovic A, Marinsek M, Svensek F. Women and men with unstable angina and/or non-ST-elevation myocardial infarction. Wien Klin Wochenschr 2006; 118(Suppl): 52-57.

[16] Kaul P, Chang WC, Westrhout C, Graham MM, Armstrong PW. Differences in admission rates and outcomes between men and women presenting to emergency departments with coronary syndromes. *CMAJ,* 2007; 177: 1193-9.

[17] Boden WE, Shah PK, Gupta V and Ohman EM. Contemporary approach to the diagnosis and managment of non- ST-segment elevation acute coronary syndromes. *Prog Cardiovasc Dis.* 2008; 50: 311-51.

[18] Thygessen K, Alpert JS, White HD, on behalf of the joint ESC/ACCF/AHA/WHF Task force for redefinition of myocardial infarction. *Eur Heart J.* 2007; 28: 2525-38.

[19] Lown B, Graboys TB: Sudden death. An ancient problem newly percieved. *Cardiovasc Med.* 1977; 2: 219-29.

[20] Killip T, Kimball JT Treatment of myocardial infarction in a coronary care unit. A two years experience with 250 patients. *Am J Cardiol.* 1967; 20: 457-64.

[21] Silber S, Albertsson P, Aviles FF, Camici PG, Colombo A, Hamm C, et al. Task Force for Percutaneous Coronary Interventions of the European Society of Cardiology. Guidelines for percutaneous coronary interventions. The Task Force for Percutaneous Coronary Interventions of the European Society of Cardiology. *Eur Heart J.* 2005; 26: 804-47.

[22] CURE investigators: Effects of pre-treatment with clopidogrel and aspirin followed by longterm therapy in patients undergoing percutaneous coronary intervention: The PCI-CURE study. *Lancet,* 2002; 358: 527-33.

[23] Jekel JF, Elmore JG, Katz DL, editors. Epidemiology, biostatistics and preventive medicine. 1st ed. Philadelphia: W. B. Saunders Company; 1996.

[24] Hasdai D, Behar S, Wallentin L, Danchin N, Gitt AK, Boersma E, Fioretti PM, Simoons ML, Battler A. A prospective survey of the characteristics, treatment and outcomes of patiens with acute coronary syndromes in Europe and the Mediterranean basin. Euro Heart Survey ACS. *Eur Heart J.* 2002; 23: 1177-89.

[25] Lindhal B, Diderholm E, Lagerquist B, Venge P, Wallentin L. Mechanisms Behind the prognostic value of troponin T in Unstable

Coronary artery disease: A FRISC II substudy. *J Am Coll Cardiol*. 2001; 38: 979-86.

[26] Rogers WJ, Frederick PD, Stoehr E, Canto JG, Ornato JP, Gibson CM, Pollack CV Jr, Gore JM, Chandra-Strobos N, Peterson ED, French WJ. Trends in presenting characteristics and hospital mortality among patients with ST elevation and non-ST elevation myocardial infarction in the National Registry of Myocardial Infarction from 1990 to 2006. *Am Heart J.* 2008; 156: 1026-34.

[27] Hochman JS, Tammis JE, Thompson TD, et al for the global use of strategies to open occluded coronary arteries in acute coronary syndromes IIb investigators. Sex, clinical presentation, and outcome in patients with acute coronary syndromes. *NEJM,* 1999; 341: 226-32.

[28] Lagerquist B, Safstrom K, Stahle E, Wallentin L, Swahn E and the FRISC II Study Group Investigators. Is early invasive treatment of unstable coronary artery disease equally effective for both women and men? *JACC,* 2001; 38: 41-8.

[29] Bowker TJ, Turner RM, Wood DA, et al. A national survey of acute myocardial infarction and ischemia (SAMII) in the U.K.: characteristics, management and in-hospital outcome in women compared to men in patients under 70 years. *Eur Heart J.* 2000; 21: 1458-63.

[30] Bennett SK, Redberg RF. Acute coronary syndromes in women: is treatment different? Should it be? *Curr Cardiol Rep.* 2004; 6: 243-52.

[31] Yusuf S, Sleight P, Pogue J, et al: Effect of angiotensin-converting-enzyme inhibitor, ramipril, on cardiovascular events in high-risk patients. The Heart Outcome Prevention Evaluation Study Investigators. *N Engl J Med.* 2000; 342: 145 – 153.

[32] Fox KM, on behalf of the EURopean trial On reduction of cardiac events with Perindopril in stable coronary Artery disease investigators: Efficacy of perindopril in reduction of cardiovascular events among patients with stable coronary artery disease: randomized, double-blind, placebo-controlled, multicenter trial (the EUROPA Study). *Lancet,* 2003; 362: 782 – 788.

[33] Marinsek M, Sinkovic A. A randomized trial comparing the effect of ramipril and losartan in survivors of ST-elevation myocardial infarction. *J Int Med Res.* 2009; 37: 1577-87.

In: Diabetes in Women   ISBN: 978-1-61668-692-5
Editor: Eliza I. Swahn, pp. 83-100   © 2010 Nova Science Publishers, Inc.

Chapter V

The Gender-Specific Impact of Diabetes on the Risk of Cardiovascular Disease

Gang Hu[*]

Chronic Disease Epidemiology Laboratory, Pennington Biomedical
Research Center,Baton Rouge, LA, USA

Abstract

The number of diabetic patients has been estimated to at least double
during the next 30 years worldwide. Cardiovascular disease is the leading
cause of death among patients with type 2 diabetes. The associations of
type 2 diabetes and hyperglycemia with the risk of cardiovascular disease
have been assessed by a number of prospective studies and the results are
consistent. Patients with type 2 diabetes have a 2-4 times higher risk of
coronary mortality than those without diabetes. Among middle-aged
general population, men have 2 to 5 times higher risk of coronary heart
disease than women. However, women with diabetes will loose their

[*] Correspondence to: Gang Hu, MD, PhD,
Chronic Disease Epidemiology Laboratory, Pennington Biomedical Research Center,
6400 Perkins Road, Baton Rouge, LA 70808
Tel: 225-763-3053, Fax: 225-763-3009
Email: gang.hu@pbrc.edu

relative protection against coronary heart disease compared with men. In recent years, several studies compared the gender specific impact of diabetes and myocardial infarction at baseline on cardiovascular mortality. These studies found that both diabetes and myocardial infarction at baseline increased coronary mortality. In women, prior myocardial infarction at baseline confers a lower or the same risk on coronary mortality than prior diabetes does. The results of these studies have important implications for clinical practice that we need to consider carefully the treatment strategies on individual disease status, particularly type 2 diabetes in women, for future coronary heart disease risk.

Cardiovascular disease (CVD), especially coronary heart disease (CHD) and stroke, is the leading killer in western societies and its prevalence is also increasing dramatically in developing nations (1, 2). Preliminary mortality data show that CVD as an underlying cause of death accounted for 34.2% of all 2 425 900 deaths in 2006 or 1 of every 2.9 deaths in the United States (3). CHD caused about 1 of every 5 deaths in the United States in 2005(3). High blood pressure, smoking, dyslipidemia, overweight or obesity, physical inactivity, diabetes, chronic inflammation, hemostatic factors, psychosocial factors, perinatal conditions and several dietary factors are the main risk factors for CVD (3-6). There is a significant difference in CVD risk between sexes (7, 8). Among middle-aged people, men have 2- to 5-times higher CVD mortality rates than women (8). The sex difference in CVD mortality cannot be completely explained by abnormal levels of conventional CVD risk factors, such as high blood pressure, lipid abnormalities, smoking and obesity (8).

Diabetes is one of the fastest growing public health problems in both developing and developed countries (9). It has been estimated that the number of individuals with diabetes among adults 20 or more years of age will double from the current 171 million in 2000 to 366 million in 2030 (9). Much of the burden of diabetes is attributable to microvascular and macrovascular complications, such as retinopathy, nephropathy, CHD, and stroke. CVD accounts for more than 70% of total mortality among patients with type 2 diabetes (10). Epidemiological studies have indicated that patients with type 2 diabetes have a 2-4 times higher risk of CVD mortality than those without diabetes (11-13). The Framingham Study is the first one to point out that women with diabetes seem to lose their relative protection against CHD compared with men (14). The reason for the higher relative risk of CHD in diabetic women than in diabetic men is still unclear. In this chapter, we summarize current results regarding the role of type 2 diabetes on the risk of CHD among women.

1. The Gender-Specific Impact of Diabetes and CHD Risk

Type 2 diabetes is associated with an increased risk of CHD, cerebrovascular disease, and peripheral vascular disease (15-18). Estimates of CHD mortality in diabetic men have varied from 1- to 3-fold of the rate in nondiabetic men (13, 16, 19, 20), whereas estimates in diabetic women have ranged from 2- to 5-fold of the rate in nondiabetic women (13, 16, 19, 20). The variation in relative risk estimates of CVD makes it difficult to evaluate the strength of diabetes as a risk factor for either sex. Several studies compared the sex-specific risk of CHD and CVD mortality between diabetic men and women.

The 14-year follow-up of the Rancho Bernardo study showed that the multivariate-adjusted relative hazards of CHD mortality in diabetic compared with non-diabetic subjects was 3.3 in women and 1.9 in men (21). An 11.6-year follow-up study in Scotland found asymptomatic hyperglycaemia (casual blood glucose > 7.0 mmol/l) to be a significant risk factor for CVD in both genders, but stronger in women than in men (22). An early review about the impact of gender on the occurrence of atherosclerotic vascular disease in type 2 diabetes reported the overall relative risk for gender (men vs. women) in CHD mortality 1.46 (95%CI 1.21-1.95) in diabetic and 2.29 (2.05-2.55) in non-diabetic subjects (23). A recent meta-analysis including prospective studies has indicated that the multivariate-adjusted summary odds ratio for CHD mortality due to diabetes was 2.3 (95% CI 1.9-2.8) for men and 2.9 (95% CI 2.2-3.8) for women (24). There were no significant sex differences in the adjusted risk associated with diabetes for CHD and CVD mortality (24). The result from DECODE study, including 8172 men and 9407 women without known diabetes, showed that newly diagnosed diabetic women had a higher relative risk for CVD death than newly diagnosed diabetic men (25). This association is statistically independent of age, body mass index, systolic blood pressure, total cholesterol and smoking (25). Moreover, in people who smoked, had hypertension, exhibited hypercholesterolaemia, or were overweight, the relative risk from CVD mortality was 1.3 to 2.1 times higher in diabetic women than in diabetic men compared with normoglycaemic women and men respectively. So we have suggested that hyperglycaemia could have a stronger additive or synergistic effect on smoking, hypertension, hypercholesterolaemia, and overweight in women than in men (25).

Moreover, most of these studies have presented the data on history of diabetes at baseline, and no study has the data on incident diabetes during follow-up. We evaluated prospectively the joint associations of history of hypertension at baseline and type 2 diabetes at baseline and during follow-up with the incidence of CHD and CHD mortality among 49,775 Finnish subjects aged 25-74 years without history of CHD and stroke (13). During a median follow-up of 21.5 years, 5074 incident CHD events were recorded, of which 3134 were fatal. CHD incidence was increased by 23% (95% CI 1.10-1.37) in men with incident diabetes during follow-up and by 90% (95% CI 1.59-2.27) in men with history of diabetes at baseline compared with non-diabetic men. In women, CHD incidence was increased by 2.04 times (95% CI 1.80-2.30) and 3.7 times (95% CI 3.02-4.53), respectively. In the joint analyses, the multivariable-adjusted hazard ratios of CHD incidence were 1.25, 1.69, 1.25, 1.83, 1.85, 2.39, 2.15, and 3.31 (p for trend <0.001), respectively, among men with hypertension I (blood pressure 140-159/90-94 mmHg or using antihypertensive drugs at baseline but blood pressure <160/95 mmHg) only, with hypertension II (blood pressure ≥160/95 mmHg) only, with incident diabetes during follow-up only, with both hypertension I and incident diabetes, with both hypertension II and incident diabetes, with history of diabetes at baseline only, with both hypertension I and history of diabetes, and with both hypertension II and history of diabetes compared with men without either of these diseases (Table 1). The corresponding hazard ratios of CHD incidence among women were 1.52, 2.37, 2.45, 3.78, 4.56, 5.63, 6.10, and 7.41 (p for trend <0.001), respectively. The corresponding HRs of coronary mortality were 1.45, 2.06, 1.08, 1.43, 1.95, 3.09, 3.08, and 4.21 in men, 1.60, 2.70, 2.90, 3.34, 5.28, 7.85, 9.24, and 10.8 in women, respectively (Table 2). Compared with men and women without hypertension and diabetes, the relative risks of incident CHD and CHD mortality were higher in women than in men with any combination of hypertension and diabetes. This sex difference was however statistically significant for only CHD incidence among subjects with hypertension I only (χ^2=4.31, 1df, P<0.05), and for both CHD incidence and CHD mortality among subjects with hypertension II only (χ^2=20.46 and 9.0, 1df, P<0.001 and P <0.005), with incident diabetes during follow-up only (χ^2=8.47 and 10.36, 1df, both P<0.005), with both hypertension I and incident diabetes (χ^2=23.16 and 17.44, 1df, both P<0.001), with both hypertension II and incident diabetes (χ^2=50.46 and 34.64, 1df, both P <0.001), with history of diabetes at baseline only (χ^2=6.02 and 4.15, 1df, P<0.025 and P <0.05), with both hypertension I and history of diabetes

(χ^2=17.91 and 14.51, 1df, both P<0.001), and with both hypertension II and history of diabetes (χ^2=16.85 and 17.07, 1df, both P<0.001).

2. The Gender-Specific Effect of Diabetes and Myocardial Infarction on CHD Risk

Another important question, whether a history of myocardial infarction (MI) carries a similar risk of CHD death as a history of type 2 diabetes does between men and women, is not fully understood. In recent years, several studies have compared the magnitude of the risk of a history of type 2 diabetes and MI on subsequent coronary mortality (19, 20, 26-32), but the results are inconsistent. The analyses from one Finnish cohort study (26) and from the Nurses' Health Study (27) found that the risk of CHD mortality among subjects with a history of diabetes without prior MI was similar to that in non-diabetic subjects with prior MI. The Health Professionals Follow-up Study (28), a Scottish population-based study (33), the Atherosclerosis Risk in Communities Study (30) and the Multiple Risk Factor Intervention Trial (31), consistently reported that the magnitudes of CHD and CVD mortality were weaker for prior diabetes at baseline than that associated with prior MI.

Six prospective studies compared CHD mortality associated with prior diabetes and established MI in men and women separately (19, 20, 29, 32, 34, 35). In the Hoorn Study, women with prior diabetes at baseline had a risk of CVD events that was similar to that of non-diabetic women with prior CVD, whereas, non-diabetic men with prior CVD conferred a higher risk of CVD events compared with men with prior diabetes and without prior CVD (34). The analysis from the Framingham Study indicated that in men prior CHD at baseline signified a higher risk for CHD mortality than prior diabetes does; however, this was reversed in women, with prior diabetes being associated with a greater risk for CHD mortality (29). In one Finnish cohort study (35), diabetes without prior MI and prior MI without diabetes indicated a similar risk for CHD death in men and women. In one large study included the entire Danish population ≥30 years of age (3.3 million individuals), diabetes without prior MI and prior MI without diabetes indicated a similar risk for CVD death in men and women, but diabetic men and women without prior MI conferred a lower risk of CHD death compared with non-diabetic men and women with prior MI (32).

Table 1. Hazard ratios for coronary heart disease incidence according to status of hypertension and diabetes (13)

	Hazard ratios (95% Confidence intervals)					
	Men			Women		
	No hypertension	Hypertension I	Hypertension II	No hypertension	Hypertension I	Hypertension II
No diabetes						
Numbers of participants	8297	7142	6531	12 587	6055	5328
Numbers of cases	612	878	1327	212	370	697
Person-years	151 508	137 660	117 205	245 868	126 333	111 157
Adjustment for age and study year	1.00	1.35 (1.21-1.49)	1.98 (1.80-2.19)	1.00	1.61 (1.35-1.91)	2.61 (2.22-3.06)
Multivariable adjustment†	1.00	1.25 (1.13-1.39)	1.69 (1.53-1.87)	1.00	1.52 (1.28-1.81)	2.37 (2.01-2.79)
Incident diabetes during follow-up						
Numbers of participants	274	444	702	291	434	778
Numbers of cases	46	117	207	31	96	249

Person-years	17 284	9862	7299	14 434	9496	6297
Adjustment for age and study year	5.32 (4.40-6.42)	4.20 (3.28-5.36)	2.86 (1.96-4.17)	2.43 (2.07-2.84)	2.25 (1.85-2.75)	1.45 (1.07-1.96)
Multivariable adjustment†	4.56 (3.73-5.58)	3.78 (2.94-4.85)	2.45 (1.67-3.57)	1.85 (1.56-2.18)	1.83 (1.50-2.25)	1.25 (0.93-1.69)
History of diabetes at baseline						
Numbers of participants	199	135	117	196	144	121
Numbers of cases	62	30	13	67	34	26
Person-years	2932	1887	1863	2413	2088	1732
Adjustment for age and study year	8.66 (6.49-11.6)	6.65 (4.51-9.80)	5.88 (3.35-10.3)	3.65 (2.83-4.71)	2.28 (1.61-3.22)	2.54 (1.71-3.76)
Multivariable adjustment†	7.41 (5.53-9.94)	6.10 (4.13-9.02)	5.63 (3.20-9.88)	3.31 (2.56-4.28)	2.15 (1.52-3.04)	2.39 (1.61-3.55)

Table 2. Hazard ratios for coronary heart disease according to status of hypertension and diabetes (13)

	Hazard ratios (95% Confidence intervals)					
	Men			Women		
	Non hypertension	Hypertension I	Hypertension II	Non hypertension	Hypertension I	Hypertension II
No diabetes						
Numbers of participants	8297	7142	6531	12 587	6055	5328
Numbers of cases	303	530	901	95	210	459
Person-years	154 598	141 929	123 140	246 859	128 163	113 835
Adjustment for age and study year	1.00	1.54 (1.34-1.77)	2.44 (2.14-2.78)	1.00	1.70 (1.33-2.17)	3.02 (2.41-3.79)
Multivariable adjustment†	1.00	1.45 (1.26-1.67)	2.06 (1.81-2.36)	1.00	1.60 (1.25-2.05)	2.70 (2.14-3.41)
Incident diabetes during follow-up						
Numbers of participants	274	444	702	291	434	778
Numbers of cases	22	55	128	20	53	183
Person-years	6527	10 283	15 548	7431	10 351	18 292

Adjustment for age and study year	1.28 (0.83-1.97)	1.82 (1.37-2.43)	2.60 (2.11-3.19)	3.49 (2.16-5.66)	3.78 (2.69-5.32)	6.40 (4.97-8.25)
Multivariable adjustment†	1.08 (0.70-1.67)	1.43 (1.07-1.91)	1.95 (1.57-2.42)	2.90 (1.78-4.71)	3.34 (2.36-4.71)	5.28 (4.05-6.90)
History of diabetes at baseline						
Numbers of participants	121	144	196	117	135	199
Numbers of cases	18	26	49	8	23	51
Person-years	1818	2155	2609	1906	1954	3100
Adjustment for age and study year	3.27 (2.03-5.26)	3.23 (2.16-4.83)	4.81 (3.55-6.52)	7.92 (3.84-16.3)	10.3 (6.49-16.4)	13.3 (9.39-18.8)
Multivariable adjustment†	3.09 (1.92-4.97)	3.08 (2.06-4.61)	4.21 (3.09-5.73)	7.85 (3.80-16.2)	9.24 (5.80-14.7)	10.8 (7.61-15.4)

* No hypertension was defined as blood pressure <140/90 mmHg and without any antihypertensive drugs treatment at baseline; Hypertension stage I was defined as blood pressure 140-159 and/or 90-94 mmHg, or with any antihypertensive drugs treatment at baseline but blood pressure <160/95 mmHg; Hypertension stage II was defined as blood pressure ≥160/95 mmHg at baseline.

†Multivariable models were adjusted for age, study year, BMI, total cholesterol, education, smoking, alcohol drinking, physical activity, and family history of myocardial infarction.

Table 3. Hazard ratios of coronary heart disease, cardiovascular, and total mortality according to the history of diabetes and myocardial infarction at baseline (20)

	Men			Women		
	Prior diabetes	Prior MI*	Prior diabetes and MI*	Prior diabetes	Prior MI*	Prior diabetes and MI*
No. of subjects	496	982	99	466	326	47
Person-years	6070	10529	859	6376	4731	479
Coronary heart disease mortality						
No. of deaths	85	320	42	74	53	17
Mortality rate/10,000 person-years†	117.3	208.5	365.9	88.7	55.6	226.3
Age and study year adjustment HR (95% CI)	1.00	1.87 (1.47-2.38)	2.93 (2.01-4.26)	1.00	0.58 (0.40-0.83)	2.73 (1.58-4.71)
Multivariate adjustment HR (95% CI)‡	1.00	1.78 (1.39-2.27)	2.97 (2.03-4.34)	1.00	0.57 (0.39-0.82)	2.26 (1.29-3.97)
Cardiovascular mortality						
No. of deaths	127	371	56	120	86	21
Mortality rate/10,000 person-years†	173.6	244.4	503.0	148.8	110.4	272.8
Age and study year adjustment HR (95% CI)	1.00	1.46 (1.19-1.79)	2.65 (1.92-3.65)	1.00	0.61 (0.46-0.81)	2.09 (1.30-3.36)
Multivariate adjustment HR (95% CI)‡	1.00	1.43 (1.16-1.77)	2.76 (2.00-3.81)	1.00	0.63 (0.47-0.84)	1.84 (1.13-3.00)
Total mortality						

No. of deaths	207	510	67	192	117	26
Mortality rate/10,000 person-years†	301.0	332.4	598.9	241.8	153.6	330.9
Age and study year adjustment HR (95% CI)	1.00	1.24 (1.05-1.46)	1.97 (1.49-2.61)	1.00	0.54 (0.42-0.68)	1.58 (1.04-2.40)
Multivariate adjustment HR (95% CI)‡	1.00	1.22 (1.03-1.44)	2.08 (1.57-2.76)	1.00	0.55 (0.43-0.70)	1.41 (0.92-2.16)

*MI=myocardial infarction; HR = hazard ratio; CI = confidence interval.

†Age-standardized mortality rate was calculated using a European standard population by 10-year age intervals.

‡Adjusted for age at baseline, study year, body mass index, systolic blood pressure, total cholesterol and smoking.

Table 4. Hazard ratios of coronary heart disease, cardiovascular, and total mortality according to incident diabetes and myocardial infarction during follow-up (20)

	Men			Women		
	Incident diabetes	Incident MI	Incident diabetes and MI	Incident diabetes	Incident MI	Incident diabetes and MI
No. of subjects	981	1308	171	1155	566	134
Person-years	6607	11215	971	9304	4646	662
Coronary heart disease mortality						
No. of deaths	102	365	47	146	126	39
Mortality rate/10,000 person-years†	150.4	301.7	506.9	123.7	190.5	496.7
Age and study year adjustment HR (95% CI)	1.00	2.04 (1.64-2.55)	3.42 (2.42-4.84)	1.00	1.57 (1.23-1.99)	4.18 (2.92-5.98)
Multivariate adjustment HR (95% CI)‡	1.00	2.15 (1.70-2.73)	3.24 (2.28-4.60)	1.00	1.65 (1.27-2.14)	3.91 (2.73-5.60)
Cardiovascular mortality						
No. of deaths	178	418	57	241	147	53
Mortality rate/10,000 person-years†	273.0	346.7	606.0	206.6	222.3	660.4
Age and study year adjustment HR (95% CI)	1.00	1.33 (1.11-1.59)	2.42 (1.79-3.27)	1.00	1.10 (0.90-1.36)	3.43 (2.53-4.63)

Multivariate adjustment HR (95% CI)‡	1.00	1.41 (1.16-1.71)	2.32 (1.71-3.14)	1.00	1.22 (0.98-1.53)	3.22 (2.38-4.36)
Total mortality						
No. of deaths	321	544	79	372	196	66
Mortality rate/10,000 person-years†	499.2	458.2	811.2	325.9	327.4	845.7
Age and study year adjustment HR (95% CI)	1.00	0.95 (0.83-1.10)	1.89 (1.48-2.42)	1.00	0.94 (0.79-1.12)	2.78 (2.13-3.62)
Multivariate adjustment HR (95% CI)‡	1.00	0.95 (0.82-1.11)	1.87 (1.46-2.40)	1.00	1.02 (0.84-1.23)	2.67 (2.05-3.48)

*MI=myocardial infarction; HR=hazard ratio; CI = confidence interval.

†Age-standardized mortality rate was calculated using a European standard population by 10-year age intervals.

‡Adjusted for age at diagnosed date, study year, body mass index, systolic blood pressure, total cholesterol and smoking.

Recently, we also compared the magnitude of diabetes and MI at baseline and during follow-up on cause-specific and all-cause mortality (19, 20). For the baseline cohort with a mean follow-up period of 12.0 years, we identified 1,119 deaths from all causes among 2,416 patients with prior diabetes and MI at baseline, of which 591 deaths were coded as CHD, 781 deaths as CVD, and 338 deaths as non-CVD. Compared with men with prior diabetes at baseline, men with prior MI had a higher risk of death from CHD (HR 1.78, 95% 1.39-2.27), from CVD (HR 1.43, 95% CI 1.16-1.77), and from all causes (HR 1.22, 95% CI 1.03-1.44) (Table 3). In women, however, those with prior MI had a lower risk of death from CHD (HR 0.57, 95% CI 0.39-0.82), from CVD (HR 0.63, 95% CI 0.47-0.84), and from all causes (HR 0.55, 95% CI 0.43-0.70) compared with women with prior diabetes at baseline. These sex differences in HRs were statistically significant for CHD mortality (χ^2=23.58, 1df, P<0.001), CVD mortality (χ^2=21.21, 1df, P<0.001), and total mortality (χ^2=29.5, 1df, P<0.001). Men and women with both prior diabetes and MI at baseline showed the highest risks of death from CHD, CVD, and all causes.

For the follow-up cohort with a mean follow-up period of 7.7 years, we identified 1,578 deaths from all causes among 4,315 patients with incident diabetes or MI, of which 825 deaths were coded as CHD, 1,094 deaths as CVD, and 484 deaths as non-CVD (Table 4). Compared with men and women with incident diabetes, men and women with incident MI had higher multivariate-adjusted HRs of CHD mortality (2.15, 95% CI 1.70-2.73 in men; 1.65, 95% CI 1.27-2.14 in women) and CVD mortality (1.41, 95% CI 1.16-1.71 in men; 1.22, 95% CI 0.98- 1.53 in women), and almost similar HRs of total mortality (0.95, 95% CI 0.82-1.11 in men; 1.02, 95% CI 0.84-1.23 in women). There was no sex difference in CHD, CVD, and all-cause mortality (χ^2=1.30, 0.59, and 0.23, respectively, 1df, all P>0.1). Men and women with both incident diabetes and MI showed the highest risks of CHD and total mortality.

Conclusion

Diabetes is a major public health, clinical, and economical problem in modern societies, and also increases the risk of CHD and CVD among both men and women. The combination of hypertension and diabetes increases the risk of CHD drastically. Diabetes and MI, either present at baseline or during follow-up, markedly increase the risk of CHD death. In men, MI at baseline or during follow-up confers a greater or the same risk on CHD mortality than diabetes does. In women, prior MI at baseline confers a lower or the same risk on CHD mortality than prior diabetes does, but incident MI during follow-up confers a greater risk than incident diabetes does. There is a gender difference of diabetes on the risk of CHD. The results of the above studies have important implications for clinical practice: First, we need to consider carefully the treatment strategies on individual disease status, particularly type 2 diabetes in women, for the future CVD risk. Furthermore, in order to reduce CVD mortality, more active management and prevention of diabetes are needed.

References

[1]   Murray CJ, Lopez AD. Mortality by cause for eight regions of the world: Global Burden of Disease Study. *Lancet* 1997;349:1269-76.

[2]   World Health Organisation. Diet, nutrition, and the prevention of chronic diseases. WHO Technical Report Series 916. 2003. World Health Organisation: Geneva.

[3]   Lloyd-Jones D, Adams R, Carnethon M, et al. Heart disease and stroke statistics--2009 update: a report from the American Heart Association Statistics Committee and Stroke Statistics Subcommittee. *Circulation* 2009;119:e21-181.

[4]   WHO Scientific Group. *Cardiovascular disease risk factors: new areas for research.* 1994; World Health Organization: Geneva.

[5]   Willett WC. Diet and health: what should we eat? *Science* 1994;264:532-7.

[6]   Thom T, Haase N, Rosamond W, et al. Heart disease and stroke statistics--2006 update: a report from the American Heart Association Statistics Committee and Stroke Statistics Subcommittee. *Circulation* 2006;113:e85-151.

[7]   Tunstall-Pedoe H, Kuulasmaa K, Amouyel P, Arveiler D, Rajakangas AM, Pajak A. Myocardial infarction and coronary deaths in the World Health Organization MONICA Project. Registration procedures, event rates, and case-fatality rates in 38 populations from 21 countries in four continents. *Circulation* 1994;90:583-612.

[8]   Jousilahti P, Vartiainen E, Tuomilehto J, Puska P. Sex, age, cardiovascular risk factors, and coronary heart disease: a prospective

follow-up study of 14 786 middle-aged men and women in Finland. *Circulation* 1999;99:1165-72.

[9]   Wild S, Roglic G, Green A, Sicree R, King H. Global prevalence of diabetes: estimates for the year 2000 and projections for 2030. *Diabetes Care* 2004;27:1047-53.

[10] Laakso M. Hyperglycemia and cardiovascular disease in type 2 diabetes. *Diabetes* 1999;48:937-42.

[11] Assmann G, Schulte H. The Prospective Cardiovascular Munster (PROCAM) study: prevalence of hyperlipidemia in persons with hypertension and/or diabetes mellitus and the relationship to coronary heart disease. *Am Heart J* 1988;116:1713-24.

[12] Stamler J, Vaccaro O, Neaton JD, Wentworth D. Diabetes, other risk factors, and 12-yr cardiovascular mortality for men screened in the Multiple Risk Factor Intervention Trial. *Diabetes Care* 1993;16:434-44.

[13] Hu G, Jousilahti P, Tuomilehto J. Joint effects of history of hypertension at baseline and type 2 diabetes at baseline and during follow-up on the risk of coronary heart disease. *Eur Heart J* 2007;28:3059-66.

[14] Kannel WB, McGee DL. Diabetes and cardiovascular disease. The Framingham study. *Jama* 1979;241:2035-8.

[15] Muller WA. Diabetes mellitus--long time survival. *J Insur Med* 1998;30:17-27.

[16] DECODE Study Group. Glucose tolerance and cardiovascular mortality: comparison of fasting and 2-hour diagnostic criteria. *Arch Intern Med* 2001;161:397-405.

[17] Hu G, Sarti C, Jousilahti P, et al. The impact of history of hypertension and type 2 diabetes at baseline on the incidence of stroke and stroke mortality. *Stroke* 2005;36:2538-43.

[18] Hyvarinen M, Tuomilehto J, Mahonen M, et al. Hyperglycemia and incidence of ischemic and hemorrhagic stroke-comparison between fasting and 2-hour glucose criteria. *Stroke* 2009;40:1633-7.

[19] Hu G, Jousilahti P, Qiao Q, Katoh S, Tuomilehto J. Sex differences in cardiovascular and total mortality among diabetic and non-diabetic individuals with or without history of myocardial infarction. *Diabetologia* 2005;48:856-61.

[20] Hu G, Jousilahti P, Qiao Q, Peltonen M, Katoh S, Tuomilehto J. The gender-specific impact of diabetes and myocardial infarction at baseline and during follow-up on mortality from all causes and coronary heart disease. *J Am Coll Cardiol* 2005;45:1413-8.

[21] Barrett-Connor EL, Cohn BA, Wingard DL, Edelstein SL. Why is diabetes mellitus a stronger risk factor for fatal ischemic heart disease in women than in men? The Rancho Bernardo Study. *Jama* 1991;265:627-31.

[22] Janghorbani M, Jones RB, Gilmour WH, Hedley AJ, Zhianpour M. A prospective population based study of gender differential in mortality from cardiovascular disease and "all causes" in asymptomatic hyperglycaemics. *J Clin Epidemiol* 1994;47:397-405.

[23] Orchard TJ. The impact of gender and general risk factors on the occurrence of atherosclerotic vascular disease in non-insulin-dependent diabetes mellitus. *Ann Med* 1996;28:323-33.

[24] Kanaya AM, Grady D, Barrett-Connor E. Explaining the sex difference in coronary heart disease mortality among patients with type 2 diabetes mellitus: a meta-analysis. *Arch Intern Med* 2002;162:1737-45.

[25] Hu G, DECODE Study Group. Gender difference in all-cause and cardiovascular mortality related to hyperglycaemia and newly-diagnosed diabetes. *Diabetologia* 2003;46:608-17.

[26] Haffner SM, Lehto S, Ronnemaa T, Pyorala K, Laakso M. Mortality from coronary heart disease in subjects with type 2 diabetes and in nondiabetic subjects with and without prior myocardial infarction. *N Engl J Med* 1998;339:229-34.

[27] Hu FB, Stampfer MJ, Solomon CG, et al. The impact of diabetes mellitus on mortality from all causes and coronary heart disease in women: 20 years of follow-up. *Arch Intern Med* 2001;161:1717-23.

[28] Lotufo PA, Gaziano JM, Chae CU, et al. Diabetes and all-cause and coronary heart disease mortality among US male physicians. *Arch Intern Med* 2001;161:242-7.

[29] Natarajan S, Liao Y, Cao G, Lipsitz SR, McGee DL. Sex differences in risk for coronary heart disease mortality associated with diabetes and established coronary heart disease. *Arch Intern Med* 2003;163:1735-40.

[30] Lee CD, Folsom AR, Pankow JS, Brancati FL. Cardiovascular events in diabetic and nondiabetic adults with or without history of myocardial infarction. *Circulation* 2004;109:855-60.

[31] Vaccaro O, Eberly LE, Neaton JD, Yang L, Riccardi G, Stamler J. Impact of diabetes and previous myocardial infarction on long-term survival: 25-year mortality follow-up of primary screenees of the Multiple Risk Factor Intervention Trial. *Arch Intern Med* 2004;164:1438-43.

[32] Schramm TK, Gislason GH, Kober L, et al. Diabetes patients requiring
      glucose-lowering therapy and nondiabetics with a prior myocardial
      infarction carry the same cardiovascular risk: a population study of 3.3
      million people. *Circulation* 2008;117:1945-54.

[33] Evans JM, Wang J, Morris AD. Comparison of cardiovascular risk
      between patients with type 2 diabetes and those who had had a
      myocardial infarction: cross sectional and cohort studies. *Bmj*
      2002;324:939-42.

[34] Becker A, Bos G, de Vegt F, et al. Cardiovascular events in type 2
      diabetes: comparison with nondiabetic individuals without and with
      prior cardiovascular disease. 10-year follow-up of the Hoorn Study. *Eur
      Heart J.* 2003;24:1406-13.

[35] Juutilainen A, Lehto S, Ronnemaa T, Pyorala K, Laakso M. Type 2
      diabetes as a "coronary heart disease equivalent": an 18-year prospective
      population-based study in Finnish subjects. *Diabetes Care*
      2005;28:2901-7.

In: Diabetes in Women
Editor: Eliza I. Swahn, pp. 101-138

ISBN: 978-1-61668-692-5
© 2010 Nova Science Publishers, Inc.

Chapter VI

Depression in Women with Diabetes: A Review and Methodological Critique

Julie Wagner and Howard Tennen
University of Connecticut Health Center, USA

Abstract

Diabetes and depression are both significant public health concerns for women. Depression is a risk factor for incident type 2 diabetes, and it also increases risk for poor diabetes outcomes. Research linking depression to health risks is limited in several important ways, particularly by common practices employed to measure depression. In this chapter we review evidence linking depression and diabetes in women, and describe limitations of the extant literature. We then review our own work that begins to address these limitations. We conclude with a review of the treatment literature and recommendations for addressing depression in women with diabetes.

Diabetes: Relevance to Women's Health

A Growing Problem

In 2005, 7% of the US population, or 20.8 million people, had diabetes. Of them, 30% were undiagnosed (Centers for Disease Control [CDC], 2005). The prevalence of type 2 diabetes is high and its incidence is rising, with a 33% increase nationwide in the 1990s (Mokdad et al., 2000). This increase can be attributed to national changes in risk-factor patterns including rising rates of obesity and overweight, an ageing population, a larger proportion of racial and ethnic minorities in the general population, as well as lower thresholds for diabetes diagnosis. Diabetes incurs tremendous economic costs. In 2002, direct costs for diabetes (such as medication and medical professional services) were estimated to be $92 billion, and indirect costs (such as lost income and disability) were estimated to be $40 billion (CDC, 2005). Approximately half the cost is spent on treatment of the metabolic condition per se, while the other half is spent on treatment of the long-term complications of diabetes. Thus, prevention of long-term complications is a primary goal of diabetes treatment.

Women and Diabetes

Changing patterns of gender and age distribution in the general population are important for understanding diabetes incidence. The greater number of women than men in the total population is the result of greater life expectancy for women in all age groups. While the female survival advantage is narrowing, greater longevity among women is projected to persist for several decades. Between 1995 and 2010, the female population is projected to grow by 17.7 million, and more than three quarters of that growth will comprise women aged 45-64 years (United States Bureau of the Census, 1996).

Women have slightly higher rates of diabetes than men. Rates of diabetes double as women age out of the reproductive years (Harris et al., 1998). Approximately 6% of women aged 45-64 years, and 13% over 60 years have diabetes (CDC, 2002) and rates are increasing (Beckles and Thompson-Reid, 2001). Older women with diabetes outnumber men with diabetes of the same age (4.5 vs. 3.7 million; Beckles and Thompson-Reid, 2001), are hospitalized for diabetes 55% more days (Aubert, 1995), and have more diabetes-related disability than diabetic men (CDC, 2000).

Minority Women and Diabetes

The US population will also become more racially and ethnically diverse over time. Population growth will rise faster for minority groups than for non-Hispanic whites. From 1995-2010, the number of Hispanic and Asian American women is expected to double, the number of African American women to increase by two thirds, and the number of American Indian women will increase by almost half (Beckles and Thompson-Reid, 2001). Minority women suffer disproportionately from diabetes; the prevalence is at least 2-4 times higher among African American, Hispanic, American Indian, and Asian Pacific Islander women compared to White women (CDC, 2005).

Classification and Prevention of Diabetes

Diabetes is a heterogeneous group of disorders characterized by glucose dysregulation including type 1 diabetes, type 2 diabetes, gestational diabetes, pre-diabetes, and latent autoimmune diabetes in adults. An important related problem common to type 2 diabetes is the metabolic syndrome which is the constellation of hypertension, dyslipidemia, hypercoagulability, glucose dysregulation, and adiposity. The two major subtypes of diabetes, type 1 and type 2, will be the focus of this chapter.

People with type 1 diabetes suffer from an autoimmune disorder which results in an absolute insulin deficiency. They require exogenous insulin for survival. Approximately 5% of individuals with diabetes have type 1 diabetes. Risk for type 1 diabetes includes a genetic predisposition and exposure to as yet unknown contagion(s) which activate the autoimmune response. Risk factors for type 1 include younger age and western European ancestry. There is currently no cure or prevention for type 1 diabetes, but promising experimental protocols include stem cell therapies.

People with type 2 diabetes suffer from a relative lack of insulin due to progressive insulin resistance and gradual loss of insulin production, with individual variation in the contribution of each. Because hyperglycemia develops gradually in type 2 diabetes, this form of diabetes frequently goes undiagnosed for many years.

Risk factors for type 2 diabetes include female sex, increasing age, genetic vulnerability, obesity/overweight, physical inactivity, and race/ethnicity, with Native Americans, Hispanics, and African Americans at increased risk relative to non-Hispanic Whites. Importantly, it is well demonstrated that type 2 diabetes can be prevented or delayed. The Diabetes Prevention Program showed that among individuals at high risk for type 2, weight loss and physical activity decreased the conversion to overt type 2 diabetes by 58% (Knowler et al., 2002), and metformin, a medication traditionally used to treat diabetes, decreased conversion by 31%.

Complications of Diabetes

Long term complications of diabetes can be categorized as those affecting the macrovascular, microvascular, and neurological systems. The majority of morbidity and mortality in diabetes is due to cardiovascular disease. People with diabetes are more likely to develop cardiovascular disease compared to individuals without diabetes even after controlling for other risk factors (Kannel and McGee, 1979). In fact, individuals with diabetes have a risk of a myocardial infarction equal to individuals without diabetes who have already experienced an infarction (Haffner, Lehto, Ronnemaa, Pyorala, and Laakso, 1998). Women with type 2 are at particular risk. Indeed, type 2 diabetes is the only disorder in which women have higher risk of coronary artery disease than men. Our work has shown that people with diabetes lack knowledge of their risk for cardiovascular disease. Women with diabetes are largely unaware of the additional risk their sex confers (Wagner, Lacey, Abbott, de Groot, and Chyun, 2006).

There are well documented racial disparities in diabetes outcomes, including among women. Mortality rates for diabetes are greater for African Americans compared to Whites, with a larger gap for women than men (Department of Health and Human Services, 1999; American Diabetes Association [ADA], 2001). Relative to Whites, African Americans are more likely to suffer some long term complications including blindness (Harris, Klein, Rowland, and Byrd-Holt, 1998), tissue injury that requires amputation (ADA, 2004), and nephropathy (United States Renal Data System, 1999). The reason for these disparities is almost certainly multifactorial, and may include genetic, physiological, behavioral, and cultural factors. African American diabetic women have higher rates of hypertension than White diabetic women (Cowie and Harris, 1995) and a worse profile of diurnal blood pressure patterns. Diabetic African Americans also have worse glycemic control than Whites even after adjustment for treatment status (Haffner, Rosenthal, Hazuda, Stern, and Franco, 1984). Relative to Whites, African Americans have poorer diabetes self care behaviors (Auslander, Thompson, Dreitzer, White, and Santiago, 1997) even when financial barriers to medication are equalized (Charles, Good, Hanusa, Chang, and Whittle 2003). As we discuss later in the chapter, depression screening, diagnosis, and treatment initiation also varies by race in diabetes.

Several well controlled trials with decades of follow up show that the risk of some long-term complications can be reduced with proper diabetes treatment. (Diabetes Control and Complications Trial Research Group, 1993; The United Kingdom Prospective Diabetes Study Group, 1998). These studies showed definitively that tighter glycemic control decreases the likelihood of long term complications. Glycemic control is measured with glycosylated hemoglobin in the blood (HbA1c), which provides an indication of average blood glucose levels over 6-10 weeks. These studies also demonstrate that blood-pressure and lipid management are important treatment targets.

Unfortunately, tight glycemic control continues to be elusive for many people with diabetes. The diabetes regimen is a complex balancing act, coordinating medication, carbohydrate intake, and physical activity. When this delicate balance is disrupted, as is often the case, short-term complications occur, which include episodes of hypo- and hyper-glycemia. There are numerous cognitive, psychological, social, and environmental barriers to diabetes self-care. Ruggiero, Glasgow, Dryfoos, Rossi, Prochaska, Orleans, et al. (1997) found that in their large sample, more than 20% did not usually self-monitor blood glucose as prescribed, nearly 60% did not usually exercise as prescribed, and more than a third did not eat according to their prescribed meal plan.

Depression in Diabetes: A Women's Health Issue

Major Depressive Disorder is Prevalent among Women with Diabetes

A major depressive episode—also referred to as major depression or clinical depression—is characterized by at least two weeks of depressed mood or loss of interest or pleasure most of the day, nearly every day. These symptoms impair the affected person's social, occupational and/or educational functioning. In addition to mood disturbance or loss of interest, the depressed individual manifests at least four of the following symptoms every day or nearly every day: significant weight loss or weight gain, motor agitation or slowing, insomnia or hypersomnia, fatigue or loss of energy, feelings of worthlessness or excessive guilt, impaired concentration or indecisiveness, or recurrent thoughts of death. Depression here is distinguished from more general diabetes distress, which is defined as patient concerns about disease management, support, emotional burden, and access to care (Fisher, Skaff, Mullan, Arean, Mohr, et al. 2007).

Major depressive disorder is common in the general population, with 17% lifetime prevalence (Kessler et al., 2004). Associated impairments (Wells et al., 1989; Hays, Wells, Sherbourne, Rogers, and Spritzer, 1995) make it the 4th most disabling illness globally (Ustün, Ayuso-Mateos, Chatterji, Mathers, and Murray 2004). Lifetime prevalence in the general population is twice as high in women (10-25%) as men (5-12%; Kessler et al.; 2004) and twice as high in persons with type 1 and type 2 diabetes as controls (Anderson, Freedland, Clouse, and Lustman, 2001). Approximately 1 in 4 people with diabetes experience major depression in their lifetime (Anderson et al., 2001). As in the general population, prevalence is higher among diabetic women than diabetic men. Women with diabetes have 1.6 times the risk of depression compared to their male counterparts, with 28.2% of women and 18% of men reporting significant depressive symptoms. Among people with diabetes, evidence comparing African Americans and Latinos with Whites suggests that rates of depression in minorities with diabetes are commensurate with, or slightly exceed that of, rates of depression in Whites with diabetes (Gary, Crum, Cooper-Patrick, Ford, and Brancati, 2000; Grandinetti et al., 2000; Gross et al., 2004). Higher rates for Native Americans have also been reported recently (Sahmoun, Markland, and Helgerson, 2007; Li, Ford, Strine, and Mokdad, 2008).

There are scant data regarding depression and diabetes in pregnancy. What data do exist suggest that pregnant diabetic women and pregnant nondiabetic controls do not differ on depressive symptoms (Langer and Langer, 1994). Additionally, women with gestational diabetes and women with pregnancy in existing diabetes do not differ on depressive symptoms. Women with gestational diabetes do show higher anxiety, though, than women with pregnancy in existing diabetes (York et al., 1996). Diabetes (gestational or pre-existing) in pregnancy usually entails an increasingly rigorous regimen, including frequent self-monitoring of blood glucose and multiple daily insulin injections. Langer and Langer (1994) showed that intensified management of newly diagnosed gestational diabetes mellitus does not increase patient anxiety and depression, and in fact is perceived as reassuring to patients. This is an important consideration, as treatment of gestational diabetes reduces serious perinatal morbidity and may also improve the woman's health-related quality of life (Crowther et al., 2004). Two studies compared depressive symptoms of pregnant women prior to and then again after being screened for gestational diabetes (Rumbold and Crowther, 2002; Kerbel, Glazier, Holzapfel, Yeung, and Lofsky, 1997). Both studies found that compared to pre-screening, women who were positive for gestational diabetes had decreased perceptions of their own health post-screening, however they showed no changes in levels of depression.

Because type 2 diabetes can be prevented or delayed, and because interventions to prevent type 1 diabetes are being tested, individuals are sometimes screened for diabetes risk. Eborall et al. (2007) investigated over 7000 individuals who were screened for type 2 diabetes. After the initial screen, compared with participants who screened negative, those who screened positive reported more depressive symptoms, although effect sizes were small. Keruish and colleagues (2007) investigated depressive symptoms among mothers of infants tested at birth for genetic susceptibility to type 1 diabetes. Mothers of high risk, low risk, and untested infants showed similar levels of depression over 1 year after screening. Similarly, Hood et al. (2005) assessed depression among mothers of at-risk infants who were identified through newborn genetic screening. For the most part, mothers of infants genetically at risk for type 1 diabetes did not report elevated depressive symptoms. This suggests that most mothers are resilient when notified of infant risk. However, certain maternal characteristics such as ethnic minority status, less than a high school education, postpartum depressive symptoms, and a history of major depression, were associated with a depressive maternal response to the news of an infant's increased genetic risk for type 1 diabetes.

Among individuals with diabetes, additional risk factors for depression include younger age, low education attainment, being unmarried, smoking, overweight, treatment with insulin, and presence of diabetes complications (Ruggiero, Wagner, and de Groot, 2006). The nature of the relationship between diabetes and depression, and any common underlying genetic, environmental, behavioral, and hormonal mechanisms have not been fully elucidated. The relationship is likely multifactorial with individual variability in the relative contribution of each factor. It is possible that slightly different mechanisms are influential in men and women. For example, Suarez (2006) investigated glucose metabolism and emotion in nondiabetic men and women. Insulin resistance and insulin levels were associatd with depressive symptoms, hostility, and anger expression among women, but not among men.

Course and Costs of Depression in Diabetes

The trajectory of comorbidity is different for type 1 and type 2 diabetes. Type 1 diabetes tends to be diagnosed prior to a first depressive episode. This is likely a reflection of the typical age of onset for the two disorders; i.e., type 1 diabetes tends to be diagnosed in childhood with average onset during puberty, whereas a first depressive episode tends to present during the second or third decade of life. In type 2 diabetes, the first depressive episode tends to occur prior to a diabetes diagnosis. In fact, prospective data show that depression is a risk factor for onset of type 2 diabetes. Taken together, the data do not support depression as simply a psychological reaction to diagnosis of type 2 diabetes, its treatment, or its complications, although this may certainly occur in some individuals.

The duration of depressive episodes in individuals with diabetes may be longer and more persistent than those documented in the general population (Peyrot and Rubin, 1999). One study of persons enrolled in a diabetes education program found that 34% of participants continued to report clinically significant depressive symptoms 6 months after initial evaluation. Relapse may also be more common, and inter-episode recovery less complete, among depressed individuals with diabetes. In a review of the literature,

Lustman, Clouse, and Freedland (1998) concluded that diabetic patients who have experienced depression are subsequently seldom free of depressive symptoms for more than a year.

Depression has a clinically meaningful detrimental association with glycemic control in persons with both type 1 and type 2 diabetes (Lustman et al., 2000). Some evidence suggests that the relationship between depression and glycemic control may be stronger for women than for men (Pouwer and Snoek, 2001). The relationship is likely bi-directional, with depression contributing to hyperglycemia, and hyperglycemia in turn contributing to mood disturbance. Depression may affect glycemic control directly via metabolic and hormonal perturbations. Depression may also affect glycemic control indirectly through compromised self-care behaviors. People with comorbid depression and diabetes show decrements in adherence to multiple components of their diabetes self-care regimen (Ciechenowski, Katon, and Russo, 2000). Some data suggest this relationship is stronger for men than women (Nau, Aikens, and Pacholski, 2007). Hyperglycemia also diminishes response to depression treatment, thus increasing risk of depression recurrence (Lustman, Freedland, Griffith, and Clouse, 1998).

Depression has also been shown to have a moderate relationship with worsened long-term diabetes complications, including neurological, macrovascular, and microvascular complications. Meta-analysis shows a consistent cross-sectional relationship between depression and macrovascular complications of type 2 diabetes (de Groot, Anderson, Freedland, Clouse, and Lustman, 2001). One longitudinal study assessed diabetic women annually for 10 years, and found that depression at baseline accelerated the development of heart disease (Clouse et al., 2003). Although depression is associated with hyperglycemia, and hyperglycemia is implicated in complications, the available evidence suggests that depression is not related to complications simply via hyperglycemia.

The costs associated with comorbid diabetes and depression are considerable, including costs for ambulatory care and prescription use (Egede, Zhen, and Simpson, 2002). Depression in diabetes also increases disability (Egede, 2004) and risk for mortality (Zhang et al., 2005). Much of the disability and financial burden of depression in diabetes is due to long-term complications.

Limitations of Previous Studies and Findings Using Alternative Approaches

Previous studies of depression and diabetes outcomes are limited by common practices in depression measurement, which influence determination of 'case' and 'control' participants in controlled studies. We now describe these limitations, the approaches used in our own program of research to address them, and the findings that have resulted from our approaches. Outcomes have included psychological well-being, self-care behaviors, medical and mental health symptoms, and markers of cardiovascular function.

The findings discussed below are drawn from our ongoing program of research which has essentially employed a 2 (diabetes vs non-diabetic) X 2 (history of major depressive disorder [MDD] vs never depressed) design to study diabetes outcomes among postmenopausal women who are not depressed at the time of their study participation. Women with type 2 diabetes (n=79) were over-sampled and compared to non-diabetic controls (n=74). Participants in the diabetes sub-sample were diagnosed on average nearly 6 years prior to study participation, with HbA1c M=6.7 indicating adequate glycemic control. Participants with a history of depression were over-sampled (n=62) and compared to never depressed controls (n=84). The previously depressed sub-sample had their first MDD episode when they were, on average, 36 years old. Forty-three percent of the previously depressed participants had a single lifetime major depression, and another 34% had experienced two or more depressive episodes. The average time since remission of their most recent episode was nearly twelve years. To be eligible for the study, individuals were required to be free of current mood disorder and antidepressant use for at least 12 months. Among the diabetic women with a history of depression, the vast majority (96%) experienced their first depressive episode prior to being diagnosed with diabetes, with an average lag time of 18.2 years. What follows is a methodological critique of the literature, and findings from our program of research that speak to the importance of addressing these limitations.

Relying Solely on Depression Symptom Questionnaires

Rates of depression vary by type of depression measurement. Studies using diagnostic interviews show lower rates of clinically significant depression (11.4%) than those using self-report questionnaires (31.0%; Anderson et al., 2001). This difference may reflect two issues. First, as Fisher and colleagues point out, most diabetic patients with high levels of depressive symptoms do not meet diagnostic criteria for major depression (Fisher et al., 2007). They assessed more than 500 diabetic patients for major depressive disorder by a structured interview (Composite International Diagnostic Interview [CIDI]), a questionnaire for depressive symptoms (Center for Epidemiological Studies Depression Scale [CESD; Radloff et al., 1977]), and on the Diabetes Distress Scale. They found that of individuals who scored above 16 on the CESD, 70% were not clinically depressed. Furthermore, diabetes distress was minimally related to major depression, but substantively linked to CESD scores. They concluded that the CESD may be more reflective of general emotional and diabetes-specific distress than major depressive disorder.

Second, there is an inherent difficulty associated with assessing depression in medical samples. Symptoms of diabetes can easily be confounded with symptoms of depression on a self-report questionnaire. For example, changes in appetite or weight may be attributable to either depression or the metabolic condition that is the hallmark of diabetes; sleep disruption may be attributable to either depression or frequent nighttime urination due to hyperglycemia; fatigue may be due to depression or glucose fluctuations. Because of overlapping symptoms, depression in diabetes is best measured by clinical interview rather than symptom questionnaire, whenever feasible. Lustman and colleagues (1997) evaluated the ability of the Beck Depression Inventory (BDI) to distinguish between depressed and non-depressed diabetic patients. The presence of depression was determined using the National Institute of Mental Health Diagnostic Interview Schedule (DIS; Robins et al., 1989) in accordance with the Diagnostic and Statistical Manual of Mental Disorders (DSM-III-R) criteria. The BDI total score, the somatic items alone, and the cognitive items alone all distinguished between groups. However, the somatic items performed less well than the cognitive items.

We use both approaches in tandem, employing self-report depression symptoms scales, and structured clinical interviews such as the Structured

Clinical Interview for DSM-IV (SCID; First, Spitzer, Gibbon, Williams, 1998). Our determination of presence or absence of mood disorder is made from clinical information gathered through the interviews. We assess symptom severity with the CESD.

We have explored the relationship between depressive symptoms and diabetes symptoms among women with type 2 diabetes. Current depressive symptoms were measured with the CESD, which assesses the presence and frequency of depressive symptoms during the preceding week. Diabetes symptoms were measured with the Diabetes Symptom Checklist (Grootenhuis, Snoek, Heine, Heine, and Bouter, 2004) which asks about the frequency and burden of 34 diabetes symptoms over the past month. In our study sample, aggregated diabetes symptoms were correlated with depressive symptoms on the order of r=.45. In partial correlation, both frequency and burden of diabetes symptoms were independently correlated with depressive symptoms. When diabetes symptoms were examined individually, those diabetes symptoms that can mimic depression, such as fatigue, were correlated with depressive symptoms, whereas those symptoms that would not likely mimic depression, such as vision changes, were not correlated with depressive symptoms. These findings underscore the importance of diagnostic interviewing to assess mood disorder so that judgment can be made about whether symptoms suggestive of depression might be better accounted for by diabetes.

Incomplete Characterization of the Course of Depression

Controlled studies linking depression to diabetes and its complications almost invariably compare individuals with current depression to those not currently depressed. This approach may be prone to the following limitations: (a) ignoring history of depression, thereby including in the comparison group individuals with a depression history; (b) failing to capture duration of exposure to depression; (c) overlooking the fact that the majority of people with a current depression have also had a previous depression, thus confounding current and previous depression; and (d) confounding depression and its treatment. Each of these methodological issues is discussed below.

History of Depression

By measuring only depression at study baseline, individuals who are not currently depressed are assumed to be free from the effects of depression. If previous depression is ignored, individuals who are not currently depressed, but who had experienced a depression prior to study baseline, may be misclassified into a group thought to be free from the effects of depression. In our program of research, we more accurately group participants by 'previous major depression' and 'never depressed.' This approach has yielded interesting findings.

Available evidence suggests that previous depression is associated with health problems that are temporally distant from the depressive episode (e.g., Fifield et al., 2001). For example, in the Women's Health Initiative, mortality survival curves for depressed and non- depressed study participants diverged over several years of follow up, indicating that the effect of depression on mortality is not necessarily proximal to depression assessment (Wassertheil-Smoller et al., 2004). Major depressive disorder is associated with cellular alterations that remain abnormal in remission (Post, 1999; Sheline, Sanghavi, Mintun, and Gado, 1992). This helps to explain why patients with a history of major depressive disorder prior to myocardial infarction have higher mortality than those who experience their first episode post-infarct (Lesperance, Frasure-Smith, and Talajic, 1996). Certainly there are state dependent depression effects which are perhaps even stronger than any effects that might be detected during depression remission (e.g., insulin resistance is worse in the presence of depression and improves with depression treatment; Okamura et al., 2000). Nonetheless, objective functional and structural changes, as well as subjective physical symptom changes, are documented after depression remission.

We investigated history of MDD and glycemic control among women with type 2 diabetes. Compared with their never-depressed counterparts, women with a history of major depressive disorder had higher HbA1c (7.0 vs. 6.5%), after controlling for confounding variables including CESD-derived current depressive symptoms.

We also investigated history of MDD and diabetes self-care behaviors among women with type 2 diabetes. Physical activity was assessed with the Framingham Physical Activity scale (Kannel, 1997); self-monitoring of blood glucose (SMBG) was measured with the Measure of Invasiveness and

Skipping SMBG (MISS; Wagner, Malchoff, and Abbott, 2005). After controlling for confounders including current depressive symptoms on the CESD, women with a history of depression showed lower physical activity scores and more frequent skipping SMBG compared to their never depressed counterparts. These findings suggest that women with a history of depression show poor self-care behaviors, even in the absence of current mood disorder and controlling for current depressive symptoms.

In examining each of these questions, had we examined only current depression, previously depressed persons who were no longer depressed would have been included with never depressed participants, increasing variance within groups, and thus making group differences more difficult to detect.

Duration of Exposure to Depression

Most studies of depression treat the mood disorder as a binary independent variable, i.e., depressed vs. not depressed, or occasionally, history of depression vs. never depressed. This approach does not consider duration of exposure to depression over the lifespan. Major depressive disorder is often a chronic, progressive condition with each episode increasing the likelihood of an additional episode, and subsequent inter-episode recovery periods of shorter duration with decreased symptom relief. Of those individuals with an episode of major depression, 41% will have a second episode within a year, 59% within 2 years, and 74% within 5 years (American Psychiatric Association; DSM-IV). Studies suggest that single episode depression may be taxonomically different from recurrent depression. For example, compared to individuals with a single prior depressive episode, those with recurrent depression manifest greater sleep disturbance (Jindal et al., 2002), memory deficits (Basso and Bornstein, 1999), and less response to placebos (Bialik, Ravindran, Bakish, and Lapierre, 1995). They also generate more stressful life events than their single-episode or never-depressed counterparts (Harkness, Monroe, Simons, and Thase, 1999). In light of this evidence, we measure the number of major depressive episodes experienced over the lifespan.

We studied the effect of number of depressive episodes on cardiovascular functioning. Flow mediated dilation (FMD) is a noninvasive measure of endothelial functioning, which is an early marker of cardiovascular disease. Diseased vessels dilate less fully; in some severely impaired vessels, paradoxical vasoconstriction can occur. Unlike the women who had experienced a single depression and never depressed women who showed similar levels of vasodilation, women with history of recurrent depression showed vasoconstriction. Controlling for confounds including CESD derived current depressive symptoms, history of recurrent depressive disorder predicted greater likelihood of vasoconstriction, but history of single depressive disorder did not. Women with single episode depression histories more closely resembled never depressed women than they resemble women with multiple episodes. These findings are consistent with a literature suggesting that recurrent depression is associated with a more severe neurophysiologic substrate and more environmental insults than phenotypically similar single episode cases (Jindal et al., 2002). Determination of number of episodes, particularly single or recurrent, may improve our understanding of who among those with MDD is at risk for poor health outcomes, including diabetes outcomes, and how MDD may confer that risk.

Current Plus Previous Depression

With very few exceptions, studies of depression as a health risk confound current and previous depression. Over the course of the depressive illness, the onset of depressive episodes may become decreasingly related to environmental adversities. This presumably results from sensitization to the state of depression, referred to as the 'kindling effect' (Solomon et al., 2000; Segal, Williams, Teasdale, and Gemar, 1996; Kendler, Thornton, and Gardner, 2000; Kendler, Thornton, and Gardner, 2001). Because the modal age of first major depressive episode is in young adulthood (Bijl, De Graff, Ravelli, Smit, and Vollebergh, 2002), this 'kindling' effect can be reasoned backwards, i.e., that a late middle-aged woman with a major depressive disorder at study baseline has a reasonable probability of having had a prior depressive episode, or numerous prior episodes. To the extent that this is the case, using baseline major depressive disorder as a predictor of health outcomes confounds 'current' major depressive disorder with 'lifetime exposure' to major depressive disorder (Tennen, Hall, and Affleck, 1995a; Tennen, Hall, Affleck, 1995b). We propose that both lifetime and current mood disorder should be considered as simultaneous predictors of health outcomes. This approach would shed light on the relative contributions of state-dependent effects of depression versus effects of accumulated exposure to depression on health risk.

We addressed this issue in a secondary data analysis of the relationship between mood disorder and coronary heart disease risk among 10,573 adults aged 60 and older from the National Epidemiologic Survey on Alcohol and Related Conditions (Herbst, Pietrzak, Wagner, White, and Petry, 2007). In the first analysis, along with covariates, past-year mood disorder predicted presence of coronary heart disease. In the second analysis, along with all covariates, both any lifetime and any past-year mood disorder were entered into the equation simultaneously to ascertain whether recency of mood disorders was more closely associated with coronary heart disease than a lifetime history of a mood disorder. Any lifetime mood disorder continued to be associated with coronary heart disease, but any past-year mood disorder was not. These data support the hypothesis that in older persons, current mood disorder may function as a proxy for history of mood disorder.

Depression and its Treatment

Many epidemiological studies that rely on medical record reviews or registry data use antidepressant use as a surrogate for presence of depression. However, resulting differences in clinical indicators between persons taking antidepressant medication, and those not taking antidepressant medication, may be difficult to interpret. Differences could be due to either depression or its treatment. In our research, we investigate depression and its treatment separately. In fact, to be eligible for our studies on history of depression and health outcomes, participants must be free from antidepressant medications for at least one year. This way, differences between previously depressed and never depressed groups cannot be better accounted for the potential effects of antidepressant medication.

Many participants, even those not currently taking antidepressants, have taken antidepressant medications in the past. We carefully assess medication history using the same measurement strategy that we employ for history of depression. Even so, findings must be interpreted cautiously. For example, in our sample of diabetic women; those who endorse a history of antidepressant use show higher diabetes symptom scores compared to nonusers. One might (mis)interpret this as indicating that a side effect of antidepressants is to cause, potentiate, or exacerbate diabetes symptoms. However, when we limit our analyses to those women with a history of depression, those who endorse a history of antidepressant use show *lower* diabetes symptom scores than nonusers, even after controlling for CESD scores. Studies that use chart reviews, registries, and other types of medical record data must be cautious in their use of treatment as a marker for disease.

Measurement of Depression

In order to address the limitations of depression measurement noted thus far, we have combined several established methods to assess lifetime depressive episodes and their treatment. At its core, our measurement strategy employs the Structured Clinical Interview for DSM-IV (First, Spitzer, Gibbon, and Williams, 1998), expanded to collect diagnostic information on every past episode.

Reliability of retrospective data is limited by participant recall and bias. Bias is most likely a problem when current mood colors recollection. For example, Aneshensel and colleagues (1987) examined lifetime history of depression in 601 participants over five waves of data collection. They found that follow-up reports of history of depression were inconsistent with reports made three to four years earlier; the predominant inconsistency was failure to report a previously reported depressive episode. The presence of internal symptom cues or external stress cues prompted recollection of past disorder. Aneshensel et al. concluded that individuals seem to alter their reports of past experience to make past states consistent with current states.

Reliability is also limited by poor recall. In order to enhance recall, we have adapted for use with the SCID, a reliable, validated, and widely used method for assessing past behaviors. The TimeLine Follow-Back (TLFB; Sobell and Sobell 1995) is a measure of past behavior widely used in behavioral studies with both clinical and non-clinical populations. The method is recommended for use when relatively precise estimates are necessary, especially when assessment of intra-individual variability is required. TLFB provides more precise information than standard questionnaires or unaided recall strategies. Our TLFB interviews include memory aids. For example, key dates and life events serve as anchors, and a visual timeline calendar is constructed with the participant to graphically represent this information (see Figure 1). By reviewing the timeline, the interviewer can assist the participant in providing a detailed picture of the time period under study (e.g., onset, duration, intensity, remission, relapse, treatment initiation and termination).

The TLFB was used in the NIH-funded Project MATCH, a multisite randomized controlled trial of alcohol treatment (Project MATCH Research Group, 1993). It has been used with adults and adolescents, men and women, different racial groups, individuals of varying educational backgrounds, the mentally ill (Sokya et al., 2003; Carey, Cocco, and Simons, 1996), both in the US and abroad (Shimizu et al., 1997; Gastpar et al., 2002). Originally designed to assess past alcohol use, the TLFB has been applied to past sexual behavior (Weinhardt et al., 1998; Midanik et al., 1998; Wickramasinghe, 1998; Crosby, Stall, Paul, Barrett, and Midanik, 1996; Stein, Anderson, Charuvastra, and Friedmann, 2001), past binge eating (Bardone, Krahn, Goodman, and Searles, 2000), past gambling (Weinstock, Whelan, and Meyeres, 2004; Hodgins and Makarchuk 2003), and past substance use (Stephens, Babor, Kadden, and Miller, 2002; Hersh, Mulgrew, Van Kirk, and Kranzler, 1999). We have adapted the TLFB to assess past depression with the SCID. To our knowledge, ours is the first application of the TLFB to psychiatric symptoms.

The TLFB has demonstrated high test-retest reliability, content validity, concurrent criterion validity, collateral (informant) validity, and construct validity in both general and clinical samples (National Institute on Alcohol Abuse and Addiction, 2004). Validity of the method is related to respondent motivation, i.e., validity is highest when the respondent is willingly engaged in the interview procedure, as participants in our study are (Vinson, Reidinger, and Wilcosky, 2003). We use the TLFB to create a visual timeline in collaboration with the participant. Such timeline construction has many benefits. First, asking research participants to anchor their memories to specific events facilitates their recall. For example, a participant may not be able to recall the date of symptom onset, but may be able recall that symptoms began 'just prior to my wedding in 1978,' or 'the week my son was born.' This is particularly true for ageing individuals and those with substance abuse, physical or emotional trauma histories that interfere with recall. Second, making differential diagnosis is facilitated by the clear outline of an individual's intertwined medical, psychiatric, and psychosocial histories. Third, people who are attempting to deceive the interviewer will have fewer opportunities to obfuscate their symptoms when they are laid out sequentially.

Traditional assessments using structured interviews such as the SCID explore clusters of symptoms at a time, jumping from past to present repeatedly, leaving both clinician and patient with a disjointed sense of events. Key information for accurate diagnosis often includes the manifestation of symptoms prior to a certain age, duration of symptoms, symptoms occurring in absence of another disorder, or the presence of symptoms in relation to life events. It can be helpful to organize disparate information into a multilayered, linear format.

We designed a timeline (see figure 1 for data from a fictional participant) to visually represent, along the Y-axis, the sequence of significant life events, psychiatric and medical symptoms and treatments, as well as subjective psychosocial functioning. The X axis displays both calendar year and patient age. An average lifespan is displayed in two year intervals with the most recent two decades (in bold) laid out annually for more detailed accounting of recent symptoms and functioning. All of these features can be modified to suit the needs of the user for a useful "at a glance" window into multiple dimensions of a complex history. In our experience, a brief explanation of the timeline to research participants is sufficient.

Our preliminary data show 100% inter-rater reliability for presence/absence of lifetime history of major depressive disorder. As would be expected, the inter-rater reliability for any individual SCID symptom is in fact lower than 100% (ranging from 60%-100%, averaging 94%). It is not unusual to have inter-rater agreement for presence/absence of Axis I disorders (including major depressive disorder) in the 'excellent' range when using the SCID (Skre, 1991). However, we attribute our unusually high reliability to our use of the TLFB, and visual timeline construction.

Why it Matters: Depression in Persons with Diabetes is Modifiable

Depression Treatment in Diabetes

Depression is an important predictor of diabetes outcomes not only because it is common and burdensome, but also because it is modifiable. Behavioral, pharmacological, and case management treatments for major depressive disorder and elevated depressive symptoms have been shown to be effective in diabetes.

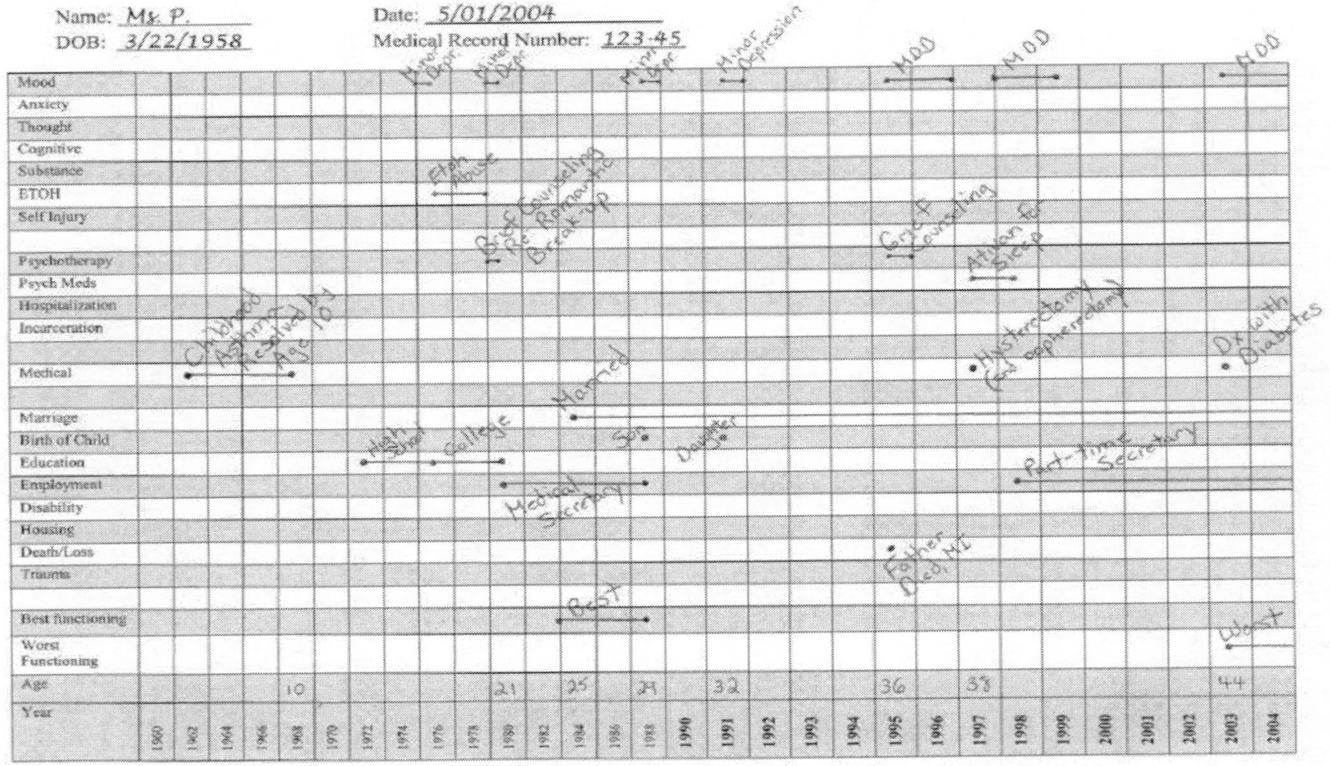

Figure 1. Visual timeline calendar which uses key dates and life events as anchors to aid recall

Available evidence suggests that when diabetes patients receive a depression intervention, whether psychological or pharmacological, they are largely satisfied with the treatment (de Groot, Pinkerman, Wagner, and Hockman, 2006). Factors related to diabetes, such as self-care behaviors, glycemic control, and weight influence response to treatment. These factors should be addressed in treatment in order to optimize treatment response. The available data regarding depression treatment response either do not address sex, or do not show differences by sex. Our knowledge of diabetic women in depression treatment is limited, but there is no indication that women respond differently to depression treatment than diabetic men.

Lustman and colleagues (1998) conducted a randomized, double-blind, placebo-controlled trial to evaluate the effects of nortriptyline on depression among individuals with diabetes. Treatment was effective at reducing depressive symptoms, and depression improvement had an independent beneficial effect on glycemic control. Improved glycemic control could not be attributed to weight change or to change in diabetes self-care. However, while decreased depression improved glycemic control, an additional direct effect of nortriptyline was to *worsen* glycemic control. Thus, while effective for depression, nortriptyline is not the medication of choice for people with diabetes.

Lustman and colleagues (2000) also conducted a randomized, double-blind, placebo-controlled trial to evaluate the effects of fluoxetine on depression and glycemic control. Participants in fluoexetine treatment showed a greater reduction in depressive symptoms, compared to a placebo group. The fluoxetine group also showed a trend toward greater improvement in glycemic control, compared to placebo-treated participants. In an uncontrolled study, Amsterdam and colleagues (2006) examined the effect of s-citalopram on depression and diabetes. After sixteen weeks, they observed a statistically significant decrease in depressive symptoms, and a marginal decrease in various indices of glycemic control. Animal studies further suggest that the selective serotonin reuptake inhibitor (SSRI) sertraline may protect, and potentially restore, counterregulatory responses that enable diabetic patients to detect and respond to acute episodes of hypoglycemia (Sanders, Wilkinson, Taborsky, Al-Noori, Daumen, et al., 2008).

In another randomized, controlled trial, Lustman, Griffith, Freedland, Kissel, and Clouse (1998) compared the effects of ten weeks of cognitive behavior therapy (CBT) to no antidepressant treatment among individuals with type 2 diabetes and major depression. A greater proportion of CBT-treated participants compared to controls achieved remission; and at 6-month follow-up, CBT-treated participants had better glycemic control. In the sample as a whole, non-remission of depression was associated with poor diabetes self-care, poor glycemic control, higher weight, and a history of previous treatment for depression. In the CBT-treated group, the presence of diabetes complications and poor diabetes self-care were independent predictors of diminished response.

Finally, the Pathways study randomized 329 patients with diabetes and major depression and/or dysthymia to either collaborative case management, or usual care (Katon, Von Korff, Lin, Simon, Ludman, Russo, et al., 2004). Compared to usual care, the collaborative care model improved depression levels and outcomes, but improved depression alone did not result in improved glycemic control. Effects were also observed for patients with multiple diabetes complications (Kinder et al., 2006). This intervention also demonstrated economic benefit. Over 24 months, patients assigned to the intervention accumulated a mean of 61 additional days free of depression and had outpatient health services costs that averaged $314 less than usual care patients. When an additional day free of depression is valued at $10, the net benefit of the intervention is $952 per patient treated (Simon et al., 2007).

Patient characteristics may influence depression treatment outcomes. Ciechanowski (2006) examined the interpersonal style of patients enrolled in the depression case management intervention described above (Katon, Von Korff, Lin, Simon, Ludman, Russo, et al., 2004). He found that the collaborative care intervention resulted in better attendance at therapy visits, more positive depression outcomes, and greater satisfaction with depression care for patients with an 'independent' interpersonal style, but not for patients with an 'interactive' style. Key components of collaborative care, including proactive follow-up and treatment adapted to the patients' preferred mode of interaction, may have provided greater possibilities for interaction on patients' terms. The investigators hypothesize that this contributed to the differences in process and outcomes for patients with a less flexible relationship style.

As mentioned previously, depression in diabetes is characterized by incomplete symptom remission and high rates of recurrence. To date, one trial (Lustman et al., 2006) has examined the effect of maintenance medication on depression relapse. Patients who recovered from depression during open-label sertraline treatment continued to receive sertraline or placebo and were followed for up to 52 weeks or until depression recurred. Among patients whose depression recurred (1/3 of the study sample), the depression free interval was longer with sertraline maintenance treatment than placebo. Glycemic control improved with depression treatment, and remained improved as long as remission was sustained, regardless of treatment.

The effects of depression care on mortality among individuals with diabetes has also been also examined. Bogner et al. (2007) performed secondary analyses on data from a prospective depression management intervention. A depression care manager worked with primary care physicians to provide algorithm-based depression care. Older depressed primary care patients with diabetes in practices implementing depression care management were less likely to die over the course of a 5-year interval than depressed patients with diabetes in usual-care practices.

Together, these studies suggest that depression in individuals with diabetes can be treated effectively. Evidence for medical and financial outcomes is limited, but growing. Antidepressant medications should be chosen prudently because of iatrogenic effects of some agents on glycemic control. To improve outcomes, the role of diabetes self-care in depression treatment should be addressed directly in the context of depression treatment.

Barriers to Effective Depression Treatment

Lack of screening is a significant barrier to detection and treatment of depression. Unfortunately, as in the general population, detection of depression in persons with diabetes by healthcare providers is inadequate. Katon, Simon, Russo, Von Korff, Lin, Ludman, et al. (2004) examined rates of detection and treatment in a large HMO population. Approximately half the cases of depression in diabetes went undetected by healthcare providers. Depression in women was more likely to be detected than depression in men. Among all of those detected, only 43% received antidepressant therapy, and only 7% received 4 or more sessions of psychotherapy. From the perspective of a healthcare provider, there are many barriers to detection and treatment. Short visit times, lack of convenient referrals, reimbursement issues, and low confidence about one's own ability to measure and manage depression may all play a role.

Furthermore, patient depression itself may interfere with a healthcare providers' ability to communicate effectively with a patient. Swensen, Rose, Vittinghoff, Stewart, and Schillinger (2008) found that compared with patients with no depressive symptoms, patients with severe depressive symptoms were more likely to report suboptimal communication across multiple domains of communication, particularly those involving interactive and patient-centered communication. Domains that were suboptimal in the presence of patient depression were elicitation of patient problems, concerns, and expectations; explanations of condition; empowerment; and decision-making. These are the interactive, bi-directional components of the clinician–patient relationship that may be crucial to detecting depression and negotiating its treatment.

Rates of depression detection and treatment also vary by race and ethnicity. We surveyed a community sample of 740 persons with diabetes attending diabetes health fairs in the northeastern US (Wagner, Tsimikas, Heapy, de Groot, and Abbott, 2007). Only half of those indicating elevated depressive symptoms responded affirmatively that a healthcare provider had diagnosed depression. Rates of depressive symptoms were similar among White, African-American, and Latino participants. One quarter of the sample endorsed physician-diagnosed depression, and among those who had been diagnosed, only 40% reported pharmacological treatment. Despite equivalent symptoms among racial/ethnic groups, African-Americans reported lower rates of physician-diagnosed depression than Whites. Those African Americans who did endorse physician-diagnosed depression reported lower rates of pharmacotherapy than Whites.

One explanation for this racial difference in pharmacotherapy may be the frequent use of alternative depression treatments, especially among minorities. de Groot, Pinkerman, Wagner, and Hockman (2006) surveyed 222 persons with diabetes about depression and depression treatment. Of those who endorsed clinically significant depressive symptoms, 19% reported receiving depression treatment from alternative healers (e.g., preachers, folk doctors), and 16% reported using herbal remedies. Twenty four percent reported receiving no treatment at all. Compared to Whites, African Americans were less likely to receive antidepressant medications, receive treatment from a mental health professional, or to report any depression treatment. These differences were evident even after controlling for sociodemographic factors. The Institute of Medicine report on health disparities (Smedley, Stith, and Nelson, 2003) suggests that when differences in outcomes are noted even when sociodemographic characteristics are equalized, the source of the difference may lie in subtle or unintended discrimination in the patient-provider healthcare interaction.

While substantial gains towards societal equity for African Americans have been made, there is still evidence of considerable discrimination against African American women. Discrimination is defined as "unfair treatment received because of one's ethnicity, where ethnicity refers to various groups of individuals based on race or culture of origin" (Contrada, Ashmore, and Gary, 2000). Racial disparities in education, income, and employment are more pronounced among diabetic than nondiabetic women (Beckles and Thompson-Reid, 2001), suggesting discrimination may be particularly relevant for diabetic African American women.

We surveyed 120 African Americans with diabetes about experiences with discrimination, depression, and depression treatment (Wagner and Abbott, 2007). We found that whereas men and women reported a similar frequency of discriminatory events, these events were experienced as more stressful to women. We also found that perceived discrimination was related to depression. More perceived discrimination was related to higher depressive symptoms, greater likelihood of clinically significant symptoms, and greater likelihood of patient-reported physician-diagnosed depression. Additionally, perceptions of discrimination within healthcare settings were associated with not taking antidepressant medication. Individuals who perceive discrimination in their healthcare system may have more depressive symptoms, but those same individuals may be less trusting of providers or the medications they recommend. Although it is true that some individuals may perceive a given situation as discriminatory while others may not, the objective nature of the stressor may have less impact on health outcomes than the event's subjective meaning (Lazarus,1978; Brondolo, Rieppi, Kelly, and Gerin, 2003).

In order to realize the benefits of efficacious depression treatment, screening must first be implemented to detect depression. Implementing pharmacotherapy for depression may be challenging among minorities and those individuals who perceive discrimination in their environment, particularly in the healthcare setting.

Conclusions and Future Directions

Rates of diabetes are high and rising. Depression is common in diabetes, especially among women. When depression occurs in diabetes, it increases risk for psychological, behavioral, and health problems. Depression may be one factor that explains diabetic women's higher rates of cardiovascular disease compared to both diabetic men and nondiabetic individuals.

Research investigating the effect of depression on diabetes outcomes has several limitations, the most important of which is an overly simplistic approach to depression assessment. Surprising data have emerged from studies that use clinical interviews rather than symptoms questionnaires, that investigate history of remitted depression, that assess number of episodes, that control for current depressive symptoms, and that differentiate depression and its treatment. Our studies of diabetic women illustrate that depression is associated with long-term health outcomes that are distal from the depressive episode. We encourage investigators to employ the strategies outlined in this chapter to assess history of depression, to establish appropriate control groups, and to more fully elucidate the relationship between depression and health outcomes in diabetes.

Efficacious treatments for depression in diabetes are available, some of which show benefits for health. However, under-detection and under-treatment of depression remains problematic, especially in minorities. Recommendations for gender-specific care of women with diabetes include screening for depression (Legato, et al. 2006). Clinicians are encouraged to screen, treat, or refer for treatment their patients with diabetes.

References

American Diabetes Association. (2001). *Diabetes 2001 vital statistics.* Alexandria, VA: American Diabetes Association.

American Diabetes Association. (2004). *Diabetes statistics for African Americans.* Retrieved April 20, 2004, from www.diabetes.org/ diabetes-statistics/african-americans.jsp

American Psychiatric Association (1994). *Diagnostic and Statistical Manual of Mental Disorders, 4th edition (DSM-IV^{TM}).* Washington, DC: American Psychiatric Association.

Amsterdam, J.D., Shults, J., Rutherford, N., Schwartz, S. (2006). Safety and efficacy of s-citalopram in patients with co-morbid major depression and diabetes mellitus. *Neuropsychobiology*, 54, 208-214.

Anderson, R. J., Freedland, K. E., Clouse, R. E., and Lustman, P. J. (2001). The prevalence of comorbid depression in adults with diabetes. *Diabetes Care*, 24, 1069-1078.

Aneshensel, C. S., Estrada, A. L., Hansell, M. J., and Clark, V. A. (1987). Social psychological aspects of reporting behavior: Lifetime depressive episode reports. *Journal of Health and Social Behavior*, 28, 232-246.

Aubert, R. (1995). Diabetes-related hospitalization and hospital utilization. In National Diabetes Data Group (Eds.), *Diabetes in America (2ⁿᵈ ed.) (NIH Publication No. 95-1468)*. Bethesda, MD: National Institutes of Health.

Auslander, W. F., Thompson, S., Dreitzer, D., White N. H., and Santiago, J. V. (1997). Disparity in glycemic control and adherence between African-American and Caucasian youths with diabetes. Family and community contexts. *Diabetes Care*, 20, 1569-1575.

Bardone, A. M., Krahn, D. D., Goodman, B. M., and Searles, J. S. (2000). Using interactive voice response technology and timeline follow-back methodology in studying binge eating and drinking behavior: Different answers to different forms of the same question? *Addictive Behaviors*, 25, 1-11.

Basso, M. R. and Bornstein, R. A. (1999). Relative memory deficits in recurrent versus first-episode major depression on a word-list learning task. *Neuropsychology*, 13, 5557-63.

Beckles, G. and Thompson-Reid, A. (Eds.). (2001). *Diabetes and women's health across the life stages: A public health perspective.* Atlanta, GA: United States Department of Health and Human Services, Centers for Disease Control, National Center for Chronic Disease Prevention and Health Promotion, Division of Diabetes Translation.

Bialik, R. J., Ravindran, A. V., Bakish, D., and Lapierre, Y. D. (1995). A comparison of placebo responders and nonresponders in subgroups of depressive disorder. *Journal of Psychiatry and Neuroscience*, 20, 265-270.

Bijl, R. V., De Graff, R., Ravelli, A., Smit, F., and Vollebergh, W. A. (2002). Netherlands mental health survey and incidence study: Gender and age-specific first incidence of DSM-III-R psychiatric disorders in the general population. Social Psychiatry and Psychiatric Epidemiology, 37, 372-379.

Bogner, H. R., Morales, K. H., Post, E. P., and Bruce, M. L. (2007). Diabetes, depression, and death: a randomized controlled trial of a depression treatment program for older adults based in primary care (PROSPECT). *Diabetes Care, 30*, 3005-3010.

Brondolo, E., Rieppi, R., Kelly, K. P., and Gerin, W. (2003). Perceived racism and blood pressure: A review of literature and conceptual and methodological critique. *Annals of Behavioral Medicine, 25*, 55-65.

Carey, K. B., Cocco, K. M., and Simons, J. S. (1996). Concurrent validity of clinicians' ratings of substance abuse among psychiatric outpatients. *Psychiatric Services, 7*, 842-847.

Centers for Disease Control (2000). State-specific prevalence of disability among adults - 11 states and the District of Columbia, 1998. *Mortality and Morbidity Weekly Report, 49*, 711-714.

Centers for Disease Control. (2002). http://www.cdc.gov/diabetes/statistics/survl99/chap2/table10.htm.

Centers for Disease Control and Prevention. (2005). National diabetes fact sheet: general information and national estimates on diabetes in the United States, 2005. Atlanta, GA: U.S. Department of Health and Human Services, Centers for Disease Control and Prevention.

Charles, H., Good, C. B., Hanusa, B. H., Chang, C. C., and Whittle, J. (2003). Racial differences in adherence to cardiac medications. *Journal of the National Medical Association, 95*, 17-27.

Ciechanowski, P.S., Russo, J.E., Katon, W.J., Von Korff, M., Simon, G.E., Lin, E.H.B., Ludman, E.J., Young, B. (2006). The association of patient relationship style and outcomes in collaborative care treatment for depression in patients with diabetes. *Medical Care, 44*, 283-291.

Ciechanowski, P. S., Katon, W. J., and Russo, J. E. (2000). Depression and diabetes: Impact of depressive symptoms on adherence, function, and costs. *Archives of Internal Medicine, 160*, 3278-3285.

Clouse, R. E., Lustman, P. J., Freedland, K. E., Griffith, L. S., McGill, J. B., and Carney, R. M. (2003). Depression and coronary heart disease in women with diabetes. *Psychosomatic Medicine, 65*, 376-383.

Contrada, R. J., Ashmore, R. D., and Gary, M. L. (2001). Measures of ethnicity-related stress: Psychometric properties, ethnic group differences, and associations with well-being. *Journal of Applied Social Psychology, 31*, 1775-1820.

Cowie, C. C. and Harris, M. I. (1995). Physical and metabolic characteristics of persons with diabetes. In National Diabetes Data Group (Eds.),

Diabetes in America (2ⁿᵈ ed.). (NIH Publication No. 95-1468), Bethesda MD: National Institutes of Health, 117-133.

Crosby, G. M., Stall, R. D., Paul, J. P., Barrett, D. C., and Midanik, L. T. (1996). Condom use among gay/bisexual male substance abusers using the TLFB method. *Addictive Behaviors, 21,* 249-57.

Crowther, C.A., Hiller, J.E., Moss, J.R., McPhee, A.J., Jeffries, W.S., Robinson, J.S., Australian Carbohydrate Intolerance Study in Pregnant Women (ACHOIS) Trial Group (2005). Effect of treatment of gestational diabetes mellitus on pregnancy outcomes. *New England Journal of Medicine, 352,* 2477-86.

de Groot, M., Anderson, R., Freedland, K. E., Clouse, R. E., and Lustman, P. J. (2001). Association of depression and diabetes complications: a meta-analysis. *Psychosomatic Medicine, 63,* 619-30.

de Groot, M., Pinkerman, B., Wagner, J., and Hockman, E. (2006). Depression treatment and satisfaction in a multicultural sample of type 1 and type 2 diabetic patients. *Diabetes Care, 29,* 549-553.

Department of Health and Human Services. (1999). *Diabetes Surveillance, 1999.* Atlanta, GA: Dept. of Health and Human Services, Public Health Service.

Diabetes Control and Complications Trial Research Group (1993). The effect of intensive treatment of diabetes on the development and progression of long-term complications in insulin-dependent diabetes mellitus. *New England Journal of Medicine, 329,* 977-985.

Eborall, H.C., Griffin, S.J., Prevost, A.T., Kinmonth, A.L., French, D.P., Sutton, S. (2007). Psychological impact of screening for type 2 diabetes: controlled trial and comparative study embedded in the ADDITION (Cambridge) randomised controlled trial. *British Medical Journal, 335,* 486-494.

Egede, L. E. (2004). Diabetes, major depression and functional disability among U.S. adults. *Diabetes Care, 27,* 421-428.

Egede, L. E., Zheng, D., and Simpson, K. (2002). Comorbid depression is associated with increased health care use and expenditures in individuals with diabetes. *Diabetes Care, 25,* 464-70.

Fifield, J., McQuillan, J., Tennen, H., Sheehan, T. J., Reisine, S., Hesselbrock, V., and Rothfield, N. (2001). History of affective disorder and the temporal trajectory of fatigue in rheumatoid arthritis. *Annals of Behavioral Medicine, 23,* 34-41.

First, M., Spitzer, R., Gibbon, M., and Williams, J. (1998). *Structured clinical interview from DSM-IV, axis disorders- patient edition* (SCID-I/P Version 2.0, 8/98 revision). New York, NY, New York State Psychiatric Institute.

Fisher, L., Skaff, M.M., Mullan, J.T., Arean, P., Mohr, D., Masharani, U., Glasgow, R., and Laurencin, G. (2007). Clinical depression versus distress among patients with type 2 diabetes: not just a question of semantics. *Diabetes Care, 30*, 542-548.

Gary, T. L., Crum, R. M., Cooper-Patrick, L., Ford, D., Brancati, F. L. (2000). Depressive symptoms and metabolic control in African-Americans with type 2 diabetes. *Diabetes Care, 23*, 23-29.

Gastpar, M., Bonnet, U., Böning, J., Mann, Schmidt, L. G., Soyka, M., Wetterling, T., Kielstein, V., Labriola, D., and Croop, R. (2002). Lack of efficacy of naltrexone in the prevention of alcohol relapse: Results from a German multicenter study. *Journal of Clinical Psychopharmacology, 22*, 592-598.

Grandinetti, A., Kaholokula, J., Crabbe, K., Kenui, C., Chen, R., and Chang, H. (2000). Relationship between depressive symptoms and diabetes among native Hawaiians. *Psychoneuroendocrinology, 25*, 239-46.

Grootenhuis, P. A., Snoek, F. J., Heine, R. J., Heine, R. J., and Bouter, L. M. (2004). Development of a type 2 diabetes symptom checklist: a measure of symptom severity. *Diabetic Medicine, 11*, 253-261.

Gross, R., Olfson, M., Gameroff, M. J., Carasquillo, O., Shea, S., Feder, A., Lantigua, R., Fuentes, M., and Weissman, M. M. (2004). Depression and glycemic control in Hispanic primary care patients with diabetes. *Journal of General Internal Medicine, 20*, 460-466.

Gu, K., Cowie, C. C., and Harris, M. I. (1998). Mortality in adults with and without diabetes in a national cohort of the U.S., 1971-1993. *Diabetes Care, 21*, 1138-1145.

Haffner, S. M., Lehto, S., Rönnemaa, T., Pyörälä, K., and Laakso, M. (1998). Mortality from coronary heart disease in subjects with type 2 diabetes and in nondiabetic subjects with and without prior myocardial infarction. *New England Journal of Medicine, 339*, 229-234.

Haffner, S. M., Rosenthal, M., Hazuda, H. P., Stern, M. P., and Franco, L. J. (1984). Evaluation of three potential screening tests for diabetes mellitus in a biethnic population. *Diabetes Care, 7*, 347-353.

Harkness, K.L., Monroe, S.M., Simons, A.D., and Thase, M. (1999). The generation of life events in recurrent and non-recurrent depression. *Psychological Medicine, 29*, 135-144.

Harris, M. I., Flegal, K. M., Cowie, C. C., Eberhardt, M. S., Goldstein, D. E., Little, R. R., Wiedmeyer, H. M., and Byrd-Holt, D. D. (1998). Prevalence of diabetes, impaired fasting glucose, and impaired glucose tolerance in U.S. adults: The third national health and nutrition examination survey, 1988-1994. *Diabetes Care, 21*, 518-524.

Harris, M. I., Klein, R., Cowie, C., Rowland, M., and Byrd-Holt, D. D. (1998). Is the risk of diabetic retinopathy greater in non-Hispanic AAs and Mexican Americans than in non-Hispanic Whites with type 2 diabetes? A U.S. population study. *Diabetes Care, 21*, 1230-1235.

Hays, R. D., Wells, K. B., Sherbourne, C. D., Rogers, W., and Spritzer, K. (1995). Functioning and well-being outcomes of patients with depression compared with chronic general medical illnesses. *Archives of General Psychiatry, 52*, 11-19.

Herbst, S., Pietrzak, R.H., Wagner, J., White, W.B., and Petry, N.M. (2007). Lifetime major depression is associated with coronary heart disease in older adults: Results from the national epidemiologic survey on alcohol and related conditions. *Psychosomatic Medicine, 69*, 729-735.

Hersh, D., Mulgrew, C. L., Van Kirk, J., and Kranzler, H. R. (1999). The validity of self-reported cocaine use in two groups of cocaine abusers. *Journal of Consulting and Clinical Psychology 67,* 37-42.

Hodgins, D. and Makarchuk, K. (2003). Trusting problem gamblers: Reliability and validity of self-reported gambling behavior. *Psychology of Addictive Behaviors, 17*, 244-248.

Hood, K.K., Bennett Johnson, S., Carmichael, S.K., Laffel, L.M.B., She, J.X., Schatz, D.A. (2005). Depressive symptoms in mothers of infants identified as genetically at risk for type 1 diabetes. *Diabetes Care, 28,* 1898-1903.

Jindal, R.D., Thase, M.F., Fasiczka, A.L., Friedman, E.S., Buysse, D.J., Frank, E., and Kupfer, D.J. (2002). Electroencephalographic sleep profiles in single episode and recurrent unipolar forms of major depression: II. Comparison during remission. *Biological Psychiatry, 51,* 230-236.

Kannel, W.B. and McGee, D.L. (1979). Diabetes and glucose tolerance as risk factors for cardiovascular disease: the Framingham study. *Diabetes Care, 2*, 120-126.

Kannel, W. and Sorlie, P. (1997). Framingham physical activity index. In M Pereira et al (Eds.). A collection of physical activity questionnaires for health-related research: *Medicine and Science in Sports and Exercise, 29,* S33-5.

Katon, W. J., Simon, G., Russo, J., Von Korff, M., Lin, E. H., Ludman, E., Ciechanowski, P., and Bush, T. (2004). Quality of depression care in a population-based sample of patients with diabetes and major depression. *Medical Care, 42,* 1222-1229.

Katon, W.J., Von Korff, M., Lin, E.H., Simon, G., Ludman, E., Russo,J., Ciechanowski, P., Walker, E., and Bush, T. (2004). The pathways study: a randomized trial of collaborative care in patients with diabetes and depression. *Archives of General Psychiatry, 61,* 1042-1049.

Kendler, K., Thornton, L., and Gardener, C. (2000). Stressful life event and previous episodes in the etiology of major depression in women: An evaluation of the 'kindling' hypothesis. American *Journal of Psychiatry, 157,* 1243-1251.

Kendler, K., Thornton, L., and Gardner, C. (2001). Genetic risk, number of previous depressive episodes, and stressful life events in predicting onset of major depression. *American Journal of Psychiatry, 158,* 582-586.

Kerbel, D., Glazier, R., Holzapfel, S., Yeung ,M., Lofsky, S. (1997). Adverse effects of screening for gestational diabetes: a prospective cohort study in Toronto, Canada. *Journal of Medical Screening, 4,* 128-32.

Kessler, R. C., McGonagle, K. A., Zhao, S., Nelson, C. B., Hughes, M., Eshleman, S., Wittchen, H-U., and Kendler, KS. (1994). Lifetime and 12-month prevalence of DSM-III-R psychiatric disorders in the United States. *Archives of General Psychiatry, 51,* 8-19.

Kinder, L. S., Katon, W. J., Ludman, E., Russo, J., Simon, G., Lin, E. H., Ciechanowski, P., Von Korff, M., and Young, B. (2006). Improving depression care in patients with diabetes and multiple complications. *Journal of General Internal Medicine, 21,* 1036-1041.

Knowler, W.C., Barrett-Connor, E., Fowler, S.E., Hamman, R.F., Lachin, J.M., Walker, E.A., and Nathan, D.M. (2002). Reduction in the incidence of type 2 diabetes with lifestyle intervention or metformin. *New England Journal of Medicine, 346,* 393-403.

Kerruish, N.J., Campbell-Stokes, P.L., Gray, A., Merriman, T.R., Robertson, S.P., Taylor, B.J. (2007). Maternal psychological reaction to newborn genetic screening for type 1 diabetes. *Pediatrics, 120,* 324-35.

Langer, N., and Langer, O. Emotional adjustment to diagnosis and intensified treatment of gestational diabetes. *Obstetrics and Gynecology, 84,* 329-334.

Lazarus, R. S. (1978). A strategy for research on psychological and social factors in hypertension. Journal of Human Stress, *4*, 35-40.

Legato, M.J., Gelzer A, Goland, R., Ebner, S..A, Rajan, S., Villagra, V., Kosowski, M., Writing Group for The Partnership for Gender-Specific Medicine (2006). Gender-specific care of the patient with diabetes: review and recommendations. *Gender Medicine, 3,* 131-158.

Lesperance, F., Frasure-Smith, N., and Talajic, M. (1996). Major depression before and after myocardial infarction: its nature and consequences. *Psychosomatic Medicine*, *58*, 99-110.

Li, C., Ford, E.S., Strine, T.W., Mokdad, A.H. (2008). Prevalence of depression among U.S. adults with diabetes: Findings from the 2006 Behavioral Risk Factor Surveillance System. *Diabetes Care 31,* 105-107.

Lustman, P.J., Anderson, R.J., Freedland, K.E., de Groot, M., Carney, R.M. and Clouse, R.E. (2000). Depression and poor glycemic control.: A meta-analytic review of the literature. *Diabetes Care*, *23*, 934-942.

Lustman, P.J., Clouse, R.E., Ciechanowski, P.S., Hirsch, I.B., and Freedland, K.E. (2005). Depression-related hyperglycemia in type 1 diabetes: A mediational approach. *Psychosomatic Medicine*, *67*, 195-199.

Lustman, P. J., Clouse, R. E., and Freedland, K. E. (1998). Management of major depression in adults with diabetes: Implications of recent clinical trials. *Seminars in Clinical Neuropsychiatry. 3*, 102-114.

Lustman, P. J., Clouse, R. E., Griffith, L. S., Carney, R. M., and Freedland, K. E. (1997). Screening for depression in diabetes using the Beck Depression Inventory. *Psychosomatic Medicine*, *59*, 24-31.

Lustman, P. J., Clouse, R. E., Nix, B. D., Freedland, K. E., Ribin, E. H., McGill, J. B., Williams, M. M., Gelenberg, A. J., Ciechanowski, P. S., and Hirsch, I. B.(2006). Sertraline for prevention of depression recurrence in diabetes mellitus: a randomized, double-blind, placebo-controlled trial. *Archives of General Psychiatry*, *63*, 521-529.

Lustman, P.J., Frank, B.L., and McGill, J.B. (1991). Relationship of personality characteristics to glucose regulation in adults with diabetes. *Psychosomatic Medicine, 53,* 305-312.

Lustman, P. J., Freedland, K. E., Griffith, L. S., and Clouse, R. E. (1998). Predicting response to cognitive behavior therapy of depression in type 2 diabetes. *General Hospital Psychiatry*, *20*, 302-306.

Lustman, P. J., Freedland, K. E., Griffith, L. S., and Clouse, R. E. (2000). Fluoxetine for depression in diabetes: A randomized double blind placebo-controlled trial. *Diabetes Care, 23,* 618-623.

Lustman, P. J., Griffith, L. S., Clouse, R. E., Freedland, K. E., Eisen, S. A., Rubin, E. H., Carney, R. M., and McGill, J. B. (1995). Effects of alprazolam on glucose regulation in diabetes. Results of double-blind, placebo-controlled trial. *Diabetes Care, 18,* 1133-1139.

Lustman, P. J., Griffith, L. S., Clouse, R. E., Freedland, K. E., Eisen, S. A., Rubin, E. H., Carney, R. M., and McGill, J. B. (1998). Effects of nortryptyline on depression and glycemic control in diabetes: results of a double blind, placebo-controlled trial. *Psychosomatic Medicine, 59,* 241-250.

Midanik, L. T., Hines, A. M., Barrett, D. C., Paul, J. P., Crosby, G. M., and Stall, R. D. (1998). Self-reports of alcohol use, drug use and sexual behavior: Expanding the TLFB technique. *Journal of Studies on Alcohol, 59,* 681-689.

Mokdad, A. H., Ford, E. S., Bowman, B.A., Nelson, D. E., Engelgau, M. M., Vinicor, F., and Marks, J. S. (2000). The continuing increase of diabetes in the US. *Diabetes Care, 24,* 412.

National Institute on Alcohol Abuse and Alcoholism.(2004). Retrieved December 16, 2004 from the NIAAA website: http://www.niaaa.nih.gov/publications/publications-text.htm

Nau, D.P., Aikens, J.E., and Pacholski, A.M. (2007). Effects of gender and depression on oral medication adherence in persons with type 2 diabetes mellitus. *Gender Medicine, 4,* 205-213

Okamura, F., Tashiro, A., Utumi, A., Imai, T., Suchi, T., Tamura, D., Sato, Y., Suzuki, S., and Hongo, M. (2000). Insulin resistance in patients with depression and it changes during the clinical course of depression: Minimal model analysis. *Metabolism, 49,* 1255-1260.

Peyrot, M. and Rubin, R. R. (1999). Persistence of depressive symptoms in diabetic adults. *Diabetes Care, 22,* 448-452.

Post, RM. (1992). Transduction of psychosocial stress into the neurobiology of recurrent affective disorder. *American Journal of Psychiatry, 49,* 999-1010.

Pouwer, F., Snoek, F.J. (2001). Association between symptoms of depression and glycaemic control may be unstable across gender. *Diabetic Medicine, 18,* 595-598.

Project MATCH Research Group. (1993). Rationale and methods for a multisite clinical trial matching patients to alcoholism treatment. *Alcoholism, Clinical and Experimental Research, 17,* 1130-1145.

Radloff, L. S. (1977). The CES-D scale: A self-report depression scale for research in the general population. Applied Psychological Measurement, 1, 385-401.

Robins, L.N., Helzer, J.E., Cottler, L.B., and Goldring, E. The Diagnostic Interview Schedule-Version III-R. St. Louis, Washington University, 1989.

Ruggiero, L., Glasgow, R., Dryfoos, J. M., Rossi, J. S., Prochaska, J. O., Orleans, C. T., Prokhorov, A. V., Rossi, S. R., Greene, G. W., Reed, G. R., Kelly, K., Chobanian, L., and Johnson, S. (1997). Diabetes self-management: Self-reported recommendations and patterns in a large population. *Diabetes Care, 20,* 568-576.

Ruggiero, L., Wagner, J., and de Groot, M. (2006). Understanding the individual. In Walker, E. (Ed.), *The Art and Science of Diabetes Self-Management Education: A Desk Reference for Healthcare Professionals,* 2nd ed. Chicago, American Association of Diabetes Educators.

Rumbold, A.R., and Crowther, C.A. (2002). Women's experiences of being screened for gestational diabetes mellitus. *Australian and New Zealand Journal of Obstetrics and Gynaecology 42,* 131-137.

Sahmoun, A.E., Markland, M.J., and Helgerson, S.D. (2007). Mental health status and diabetes among Whites and Native Americans: is race an effect modifier? *Journal of Health Care for the Poor and Underserved, 18,* 599-608.

Sanders, N.M., Wilkinson, C.W., Taborsky, G.J., Al-Noori, S., Daumen, W., Zavosh, A., Figlewicz, D.P. (2008). The selective serotonin reuptake inhibitor sertraline enhances counterregulatory responses to hypoglycemia. *American Journal of Physiolical Endocrinology and Metabolism, 294,* E853-60.

Segal, Z., Williams, J., Teasdale J., and Gemar, M. (1996). A cognitive science perspective on kindling and episode sensitization in recurrent affective disorder. *Psychological Medicine, 26,* 371-180.

Sheline, Y. I., Sanghavi, M., Mintun, M. A., and Gado M. H.(1999). Depression duration but not age predicts hippocampal volume loss in medically healthy women with recurrent major depression. *Journal of Neuroscience, 19,* 5034-5043

Shimizu. S., Ito, N., Fujiwara, M., Takanashi, K., Weerakoon, S., Deshapriya, E. B. (1997). Is the TLFB method applicable to Japanese drinking population?: Methodological study on measurement of alcohol consumption. *Nihon Arukoru Yakubutsu Igakkai Zasshi, 32,*163-181.

Simon, G. E., Katon, W. J., Lin, E. H., Rutter, C., Manning, W. G., Von Korff, M., Ciechanowski, P., Ludman, E. J., and Young, B. A. (2007). Cost-effectiveness of systematic depression treatment among people with diabetes mellitus. *Archives of General Psychiatry, 64,* 65-72.

Skre, I. (1991). High interrater reliability for the Structured Clinical Interview for DSM Axis 1. *Acta Psychiatrica Scandinavica, 84,* 167-173.

Smedley, B. D., Stith, A. Y., Nelson, A. R. (Eds.). (2003). *Unequal treatment: Confronting racial and ethnic disparities in health care.* Washington, DC, National Academies Press.

Sobell, L. and Sobell, M. (1995). *Alcohol timeline followback user's manual.* Toronto, ON: Addiction Research Foundation.

Solomon, D., Keller, M., Leon, A., Mueller, T. I., Lavori, P. W., Shea, M. T., Coryell, W., Warshaw, M., Turvey, C., Maser, J. D., and Endicott, J. (2000). Multiple recurrences of major depressive disorder. *American Journal of Psychiatry, 157,* 229-233.

Soyka, M., Aichmüller C., v Bardeleben, U., Beneke, M., Glaser, T., Hornung-Knobel, S., Wegner, U. (2003). Flupenthixol in relapse prevention in schizophrenics with comorbid alcoholism. *European Addition Research, 9,* 65-72.

Stein M. D., Anderson, B., Charuvastra A., and Friedmann, P. D. (2001). Alcohol use and sexual risk taking among hazardously drinking drug injectors who attend needle exchange. *Alcoholism, Clinical and Experimental Research, 25,* 1487-1493.

Stephens, R. S., Babor, T. F., Kadden, R., and Miller, M. (2002). The marijuana treatment project: Rationale, design and participant characteristics. Addiction, 97(S1), 109-124.

Suarez, E.C. (2006). Sex differences in the relation of depressive symptoms, hostility, and anger expression to indices of glucose metabolism in nondiabetic adults. Health Psychology, 25, 484-92.

Swenson, S.L., Rose, M., Vittinghoff, E., Stewart, A., Schillinger, D. (2008). The influence of depressive symptoms on clinician-patient communication among patients with type 2 diabetes. Medical Care, 46, 257-65.

Tennen, H., Eberhardt, T., and Affleck, G. (1999). Depression research methodologies at the social-clinical interface: Still hazy after all these years. *Journal of Social and Clinical Psychology, 18*, 121-159.

Tennen, H., Hall, J., and Affleck, G. (1995a). Depression research methodologies in Journal of Personality and Social Psychology: A review and critique. *Journal of Personality and Social Psychology, 68*, 870-884.

Tennen, H., Hall, J., and Affleck, G. (1995b). Rigor, rigor mortis, and conspiratorial views of depression research. *Journal of Personality and Social Psychology, 68*, 895-900.

United Kingdom Prospective Diabetes Study (UKPDS)Group (1998). Intensive blood-glucose control with sulphonylureas or insulin compared with conventional treatment and risk of complications in patients with type 2 diabetes. *Lancet, 12*, 837-53.

United States Bureau of the Census. (1996). Population projections of the United States by age, sex, race, and Hispanic origins: 1995 to 2050. Current Population Reports, Series P25, No. 1130. Washington DC: US Government Printing Office.

United States Renal Data System. (1999). *USRDS 1999 Annual Data Report*, NIH, NIDDK, Bethesda MD 1999; CDCP, Division of Diabetes Translation: ESRD.

Üstün, T. B., Ayuso-Mateos, J. L., Chatterji, S., Mathers, C., and Murray, C. J. (2004). Global burden of depressive disorders in the year 2000. *British Journal of Psychiatry, 184*, 386-392.

Vinson, D., Reidinger, C., and Wilcosky, T. (2003). Factors affecting the validity of a TLFB interview. *Journal of Studies on Alcohol ,64*, 733-740.

Wagner, J. and Abbott, G. (2007). Depression and depression care in diabetes: Relationship to perceived discrimination in African Americans. *Diabetes Care, 30*, 364-366.

Wagner, J., Lacey, K., Abbott, G., de Groot, M., and Chyun, D. (2006). Knowledge of heart disease risk in a multicultural community sample of people with diabetes. *Annals of Behavioral Medicine, 31*, 224-230.

Wagner, J., Malchoff, C., and Abbott, G. (2005). Invasiveness as a barrier to self-monitoring of blood glucose in people with diabetes. *Diabetes Technology and Therapeutics, 7*, 612-619.

Wagner, J. and Tennen, H. (2007). History of major depressive disorder and diabetes outcomes among diet and tablet treated postmenopausal women: A case control study. *Diabetic Medicine, 24*, 211-216.

Wagner, J., Tennen, H., Mansoor, G., and Abbott, G. (in press). Endothelial dysfunction and history of depression in post-menopausal women with type 2 diabetes: A case control study. *Journal of Diabetes and its Complications*.

Wagner, J., Tsimikas, J., Heapy, A., de Groot, M., and Abbott, G. (2007). Ethnic and racial differences in diabetic patients' depressive symptoms, diagnosis, and treatment. *Diabetes Research and Clinical Practice, 75*, 119-122.

Wassertheil-Smoller, S., Shumaker, S., Ockene, J., Talavera, G. A., Greenland, P., Cochrane, B., Robbins, J., Aragaki, A., and Dunbar-Jacob J. (2—4). Depression and cardiovascular sequelae in postmenopausal women. The Women's Health Initiative (WHI). *Archives of Internal, 164*, 289-298.

Weinhardt, L. S., Carey, M. P., Maisto, S. A., Carey, K. B., Cohen, M. M., and Wickramasinghe, S. M. (1998). Reliability of the timeline follow-back sexual behavior interview. *Annals of Behavioral Medicine, 20*, 25-30.

Weinstock, J., Whelan, J. P. and Meyers, A. W. (2004). Behavioral assessment of gambling: an application of the TLFB method. *Psychological Assessment, 16*, 72-80.

Wells, K. B., Stewart, A., Hays, R. D., Burnam, M. A., Rogers, W., Daniels, M., Berry, S., Greenfield, S., and Ware, J. (1989). The functioning and well-being of depressed patients: results from the medical outcomes study. *Journal of the American Medical Association, 262*, 914-919.

Wickramasinghe, S. (1998). Reliability of the timeline follow-back sexual behavior interview. *Annals of Behavioral Medicine, 20*, 25-30.

York, R., Brown, L.P., Persily, C.A., Jacobsen, B.S. (1996). Affect in diabetic women during pregnancy and postpartum. *Nursing Research, 45*, 54-6.

Zhang, X., Norris, S. L., Gregg, E. W., Cheng, Y. J., Beckles, G., and Kahn, H. S. (2005). Depressive symptoms and mortality among persons with and without diabetes. *American Journal of Epidemiology, 161*, 652-660.

Index